STEROIDS

STEROIDS

BY HANK NUWER

Franklin Watts 1990
New York / London / Toronto / Sydney
An Impact Book

For Teresa Nuwer

Photographs courtesy of:
UPI/Bettmann Newsphotos: pp. 13, 14, 24, 26, 33, 39, 41, 46, 51, 52,
70, 85; Dave Black, 1990: pp. 28, 37, 55; AP/Wide World: pp. 58, 94;
Photo Researchers: pp. 66 (Renee Lynn), 101 (Spencer Grant); Reuters/
Bettmann Newsphotos: p. 74; Gamma-Liaison: p. 100 (Alexis Duclos).

Library of Congress Cataloging-in-Publication Data

Nuwer, Hank.
Steroids/Hank Nuwer.
p. cm.—(Impact book)
Summary: Examines the sources, uses, and effects
of steroids in sports and society.
Includes bibliographical references.
ISBN 0-531-10946-1
1. Doping in sports. 2. Anabolic steroids   Health aspects.
[1. Steroids. 2. Doping in sports.] 1. Title. II. Series.
RC1230.N88   1990
362.29 dc20   90-32757 CIP AC

Also by Hank Nuwer:

Recruiting in Sports

Strategies of the Great Baseball Managers

Strategies of the Great Football Coaches

CONTENTS

STEROIDS

1

JUST THE FACTS

A Competitive
Edge for a Price

The scene in Seoul, South Korea, was one that Canadian sprinter Ben Johnson would take to his grave. Hundreds of sportswriters, television crew members, and curious spectators had gathered together to hear the announcement that would shatter Johnson's reputation. In one brief moment, the athlete's world turned upside down. From Canada's new national hero, he had become a national disgrace. The announcement was as bad as it could be. The International Olympic Committee (IOC) said that Ben Johnson had broken regulations by taking performance-enhancing drugs. He would have to forfeit his treasured gold medal in the 100-meter event. He left South Korea in disgrace, hiding his face from photographers who were as eager to film his shame as they had his glory.

What a far cry from three days earlier! In front of 70,000 cheering fans, Ben Johnson had soundly whipped the seven fastest runners in the world, including his arch-rival, Carl Lewis. His time was 9.79, an improvement over his own 9.83 record that had earlier seemed so amazing. Lewis was .13 of a second behind Johnson, and the Canadian had even slowed slightly at the finish line to taunt him by raising his right fist to the sky in triumph.

Johnson's fall from grace intrigued the world. The revelation that he had used chemicals to gain an unfair advantage was an indication that many other athletes might also be cheating to win.

In our competitive times, people often look for an edge over the opposition. This is as true in athletics as it is in business. Athletes will try anything to win—a better diet, a better protein supplement, better-made footwear, better training methods, or better coaching. Moreover, because of the glut of physical-fitness magazines, videos, and television coverage, what one athlete discovers today in Oregon will be known tomorrow by athletes in Rhode Island and New York.

This is precisely why it is estimated by sports-medicine researcher W. N. Taylor that up to 1 million athletes and nonathletes from junior high school age to adulthood are using steroids in significant doses for extended periods of time. Young athletes have heard and seen that established athletes whom they admire have used them, and they want to follow the same victorious path their heroes have trod. Or they are certain that the competition is on steroids, and they take them to achieve parity. "I broke the rules, but I didn't gain an unfair edge over my competitors," said Duncan Atwood, a javelin thrower once suspended for steroid use who facetiously claimed he had to compete against fellow throwers who were "glowing in the dark" from drugs.[1]

Of course, talk like Atwood's is mere rationalization to justify his own actions. Make no mistake about it: To use steroids is to cheat with a capital C, and athletes fool

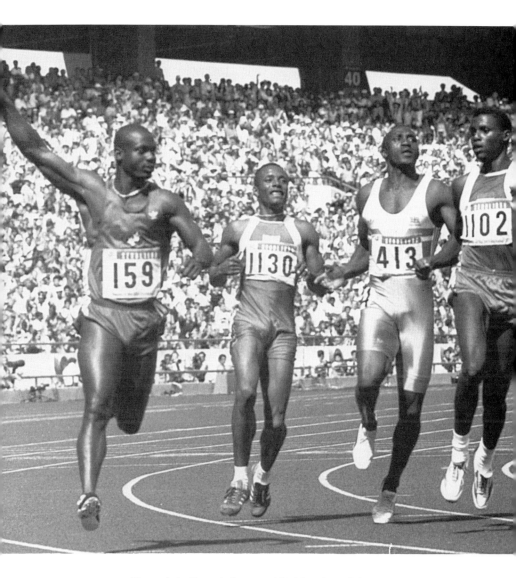

Canada's Ben Johnson (159) raises his arm in triumph after setting a new world record of 9.79 seconds in the 100-meter race September 24, 1988, at the Seoul, South Korea, Olympics.

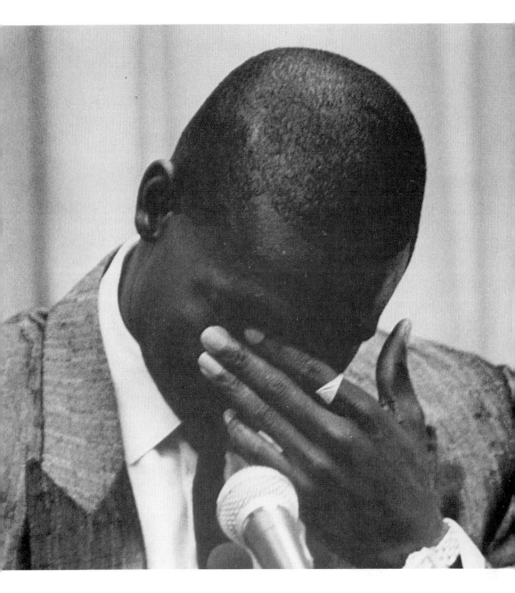

Ben Johnson wipes away tears after admitting that his denials of drug use were lies during his testimony to the Dubin Inquiry in Toronto, June 13, 1989.

no one—except maybe themselves—when they say they're only keeping abreast of the competition.

If they are not cheating, why would they take substances to mask steroid use? Why would they hide their usage from coaches and family? Why would they plan their taking of steroids to allow the substances to drain from their bodies in time to pass drug tests?

What Are Steroids?

Simply stated, steroids in nature are compounds that are necessary for the well-being of many living creatures, including human beings. These include sex hormones, bile acids, and cholesterol. The compounds perform such essential body functions as:

Regulating the balance of internal salt and water

Digesting fats

Causing the development of secondary sex characteristics, such as body hair, a deep male voice, breasts on women.[2]

Steroids certainly do have important medical purposes. They are used by doctors to help patients with anemia, burns, asthma, anorexia, cancer, hypogonadism, micropenis (in young children), and intestinal disorders and to stimulate puberty when nature fails to do so. More commonly, people take a form of steroid hormone popularly called cortisone (a glucocorticoid [glu-ko-kór-ti-koyd]) to combat hay fever.

"Cortical" steroids are not the controversial steroids that cause so much hope and heartbreak in sports and society today. Cortical steroids, or corticosteroids, include a variety of hormones that are found in the cortex (the area around the center) of the two adrenal glands (located atop the two kidneys). Cortical steroids, drugs

15

prescribed by doctors, are produced naturally and synthetically and are used to combat the effects of advanced cases of arthritis, asthma, adrenal deficiency, and other ailments.[3]

Nor is female sex hormone, known as estrogen, a problem drug. Athletes and fitness freaks certainly do not want to develop female characteristics that would be a liability in competition (although female hormones are found in some varieties of anabolic steroids).

What is desired (although not in the body's best interest) by both male and female athletes is testosterone, the male sex hormone, which accounts for the secondary sex characteristics that make men leaner, more muscular, more aggressive, and able to train harder and recover faster from intense workouts. The American College of Sports Medicine also believes that steroids can increase bone density; other researchers say they enhance muscle contractility, heal muscles faster after a workout, and cause nitrogen retention.[4] Chemists—both legally and illegally—can develop compounds of male sex hormone.

The performance enhancers that are the choice of cheating champions are androgenic-anabolic steroids—most commonly called steroids, or 'roids, by users.[5]

The word *androgenic* refers to any substance that gives rise to masculine characteristics. The term *anabolic* refers to a substance that creates protein and stimulates tissue growth. One of the myths about anabolic steroids is that they can assist in the rehabilitation of knee injuries. Both the team physician for the New England Patriots, Bertram Zarina, M.D., and the National Collegiate Athletic Association (NCAA) director of research and sports science, Ursula Walsh, have insisted that anabolic steroids have no value in the treatment of such injuries.

Many types of anabolic steroids are not allowed by amateur and professional sports federations, and many more are discovered each year. Athletes connected to underground sources say there are several others that authorities have not yet learned to locate by testing. But such stories may be nothing more than wishful thinking by athletes. Indeed, the most sophisticated users of chemicals were said to be the Bulgarians. Yet, during the 1988 Olympic Games, two gold-medal-winning weight lifters from Bulgaria were detected using steroids. Their fate was the same that befell Ben Johnson. Nonetheless, athletes persist in believing there are undetectable substances floating around in their opponents' bloodstreams.

Among the most popular chemical substances are Nelvar and Deca-Durabolin, anabolic steroids that contain natural derivatives of testosterone. Another steroid is Anavar, which is said to cause muscular definition and hardening.[6] Winstrol, a brand-name steroid also called Stanozolol, is also popular among athletes. Other popular steroids are Dianabol and Anadrol-50.

Steroid users are sophisticated consumers. They order anabolic steroids that suit their specific needs (greater body mass, better definition, bigger biceps, better time in sprints) and that also pass through the body in the shortest time possible so as to escape detection in drug tests.

Do Steroids Work?

The evidence indicates to most legitimate researchers that steroids can enhance muscle gains and athletic performance. "If steroids did not give the user a competitive edge, we would not have the problem," said researcher Charles E. Yesalis of Penn State University, who estimates that up to a half million children and adolescents alone have tried anabolic steroids.[7]

Those who feel that steroids cannot give athletes an edge are a small minority. Dr. Marcus Reidenberg, for example, a New York Hospital–Cornell Medical Center professor of pharmacology, told *Newsweek* in 1988 that he doesn't believe steroids provide strength and performance enhancement. "They may act on the brain to increase aggressiveness, which may drive an athlete to train harder and eat more," he said. "But athletes who use them to build muscle may be deceiving themselves."[8]

However, experts on steroids, such as Michael A. Nelson, M.D., insist that physicians who deny that steroids promote growth and enhance performance are the ones who are deceiving themselves. Moreover, they are doing a major disservice to users.

"For years health care professionals took the position that androgenic-anabolic steroids were not effective in promoting strength. It is clear now that that was an erroneous position," said Dr. Nelson, who has also chastised doctors who claim that steroids are not physically addicting. "Our refusal in the past to admit that [they] are effective has seriously jeopardized our legitimacy among athletes."[9]

What Dr. Reidenberg is overlooking or downplaying, moreover, is that to this day the number of serious, scientifically controlled studies on steroids has been abysmally low. Research on hormones (both those naturally produced by the body and those taken in pill or injected form) and their effect on the human body is skimpy except in the area of reproduction—and especially in regard to physical and mental performance.

Why? For one thing, scientists believe it is ethically wrong to administer steroids to human beings when all evidence indicates that some of the subjects will suffer grave bodily harm. Even those who might not have such compunctions fear lawsuits from subjects should they suffer, for example, liver damage. Society no longer tolerates giving questionable chemicals or drugs to students or prison inmates. Scientists learned many hard and unfortunate lessons earlier in this century from gov-

18

ernment experiments such as one in which the hallucinogen LSD was given volunteers, including writer Ken Kesey, and another in the Deep South in which placebos were given prisoners who suffered from syphilis.

Eventually, however, scientists and medical researchers will have much to tell us about steroids and their effects. Ironically, and sadly, the rise in the number of athletes who report physical ailments such as cancer and liver damage after prolonged steroid use will help researchers learn more about the substance. These athletes, in effect, will have turned themselves into unwitting human guinea pigs. What is not known at this early date is whether athletes using steroids who have not reported adverse effects will escape serious physical consequences. Will they continue to lead normal, productive lives, or will their lives be shortened and their later years plagued by such ailments as cancer or liver traumas? Only time can answer such speculative questions.

However, many medical experts have drawn the conclusion that the long-term use of anabolic steroids will probably harm such users. This is why drug testing of athletes in the United States is being instituted from the high school level on up to professional and top-level amateur sports. Supporting that conclusion is the recent reporting of a rash of health problems by athletes who have just now begun to suffer ailments as a result of steroid use in the seventies or early eighties.

The most visible of the athletes is Steve Courson, the former Pittsburgh Steeler and Tampa Bay Buccaneer football player. He has appeared on many television news specials and has visited high schools across the United States, speaking against the use of chemical substances that he claims have robbed him of his health. At this writing, he is hoping to receive a donor heart to replace his own, which his doctors believe has been irreversibly damaged by illicit steroid use. His message to young people is twofold: (1) "Things are not what they're always made out to be," he tells youngsters, adding that playing in the National Football League (NFL) was not worth the price in agony he is now paying. (2) "Be true to yourself." He urges youngsters not to let peer pressure sway them into building better exterior bodies at the expense of internal organs.

Courson's rejection of steroids supports the conclusions of medical experts. Just as everything in life has a price, so, too, do anabolic steroids. Those experts believe that people who indulge in them risk paying dearly for whatever rewards they may bring.

Lake Central High School (Illinois) football coach Elmer Britton said he tells his players not to use anabolic steroids because they can cause irreversible bodily damage, but he doesn't mislead his team, either. "While you realize that steroids are bad and can kill you," he said, "you have to also realize that steroids do work."[10]

Proponents of steroid use say that immediate gains are visible with steroids, and their claims are hard to dispute.

One Indiana-based peddler claims that his customers can see up to a twenty-pound gain in two months with Dianabol and up to twenty-five pounds with Anadrol-50.

This same dealer tells his buyers to take steroids in cycles. He advises them to use steroids for six to eight weeks, and then quit for two weeks while substituting human chorionic gonadotropin (HCG), a drug that he claims (many researchers disagree) stimulates the body's normal processes (such as testosterone production).[11]

Other research shows that nearly all serious steroid users take them in similar cycles. Moreover, few take just one type of steroid. Most take combinations of as many as five different brands of steroids (a process known as "stacking"), with little or no knowledge of how these drugs react with one another in combination.

Cycles vary from six to ten weeks. Many users take doses that far exceed the dosages even the most unscrupulous doctor would ever prescribe, because the athletes believe that they'll get more impressive results from larger doses.[12]

In the previously mentioned situation involving former pro-football player Steve Courson, he admitted in 1985 to taking horrendous dosages of steroids as he tried to hold on to his playing career for a season longer. "On my first eight-week cycle I did anabolics in doses of descending order," Courson told *Sports Illustrated.* "I took Winstrol, that's an oral. I took Anovar, another oral. I took Deca-Durabolin, an injectable. I took the orals every day. I injected once or twice a week."

Courson admitted that he took 300 mg (milligrams) of Deca-Durabolin in weeks one and two of the cycle. When legally prescribed by doctors for medical reasons, *the manufacturer's recommended dosage is 50–100 mg per month or three weeks.*

Courson took 50 mg a day of Winstrol. *The manufacturer's recommended dosage for patients taking the drug for medical purposes only is 6 mg daily.*

He also swallowed 50 mg a day of Anavar. *The recommended dosage for legitimate medical reasons is 5–10 mg daily.*[13]

Now, four years after the *Sports Illustrated* interview, Courson is a doomed man unless he can find a heart donor. Walking down a flight of stairs is too much exertion for a man whose goal was, in 1985, to dead-lift 1,000 pounds and bench-press 600 pounds.

Those who desire greater strength, endurance, size, and body definition believe that this edge can be obtained easily and quickly by taking anabolic steroids. These fast-acting compounds (both the natural or synthetic chemical equivalents of testosterone, the male hormone) are regarded by many male and female athletes today as their key to glory and riches. These anabolic steroids are also used by males from preteens to adults who do not compete in sports but who want to possess bodies that they believe will make them the envy of their peers.

The typical buyer of steroids is an "insecure" individual "seeking acclaim and rewards," claimed former British Olympic sprinter David Jenkins, who ought to know, since he was arrested on a steroid-related charge. "They come from a gym environment, where a muscle mentality pervades and creates a demand for bigger bench-presses, bigger squats. But they would rather not take a long-term approach. They want steroid McDonald's."[14]

At least one college football player agrees with that statement, admitting that he took steroids because he feared failure. "In my case I was a small lineman, so I could either spend time on the bench or [take them]," Tommy Chaikin, a former college football player at the University of South Carolina, told the *Los Angeles Times*. "You'll go to any lengths. You lose perspective on right and wrong. It's what drives anyone to success. . . . It becomes an ego thing. You think you become godlike, invincible."[15]

Thus, far from being a "big city" issue, steroids now are being used in remote hamlets and towns from Alaska to Florida as well as in every country in the world where athletic competition is taken seriously—some say *too* seriously.

As will be shown in more detail later, those who rely on anabolic steroids are choosing to risk short- and long-term health damage in return for immediate rewards. In other words, users may not be selling their souls for success, but they must be aware that some steroid users have sacrificed their livers or other organs. Steroids to date have not been directly shown to have caused any deaths, but as will be seen in chapter 5, they have been *linked* to dozens of deaths.

The Public Perception

The general public has recently begun to look down upon steroid users, and so those who use steroids usually have only other users, or maverick coaches and trainers, to go to for moral support of their practice. This was not always the case. In a 1984 interview I conducted with the then head coach of the San Francisco 49ers, Bill Walsh, he spoke out against drug users but cautioned that steroid users should not be lumped together with those who abuse street drugs such as cocaine.

Before he retired, however, Walsh publicly expressed his disgust for rampant steroid abuse, reporting that he'd heard players would have their own steroid-laced urine removed by catheter before a test, then have urine from "clean" teammates pumped into their own bladders.

A few years ago, Brian Bosworth, after being suspended from college bowl competition because he failed a steroid drug test, was hired for a national deodorant commercial after signing a professional contract. For a while he sent a powerful message that drug use can make you not only a better athlete, but a rich and famous one to boot. But with the fall of Olympian Ben Johnson as well as recent state and national legislation making steroid use or trafficking a crime, no respectable Madison Avenue ad agency ever again will present an acknowledged steroid user in a commercial.

"You have 'The Boz' [Bosworth] getting busted for steroids, and he's a hero in this country," scoffed long-distance runner Steve Scott. "He gets caught, and he's a freakin' hero. What sense can be made of that?"[16]

Recent public opinion polls are divided as to whether steroid use is as serious as the use of such street drugs as marijuana, cocaine, and amphetamines. What is certain, however, is that many dealers who peddle so-called street drugs now have decided that selling ste-

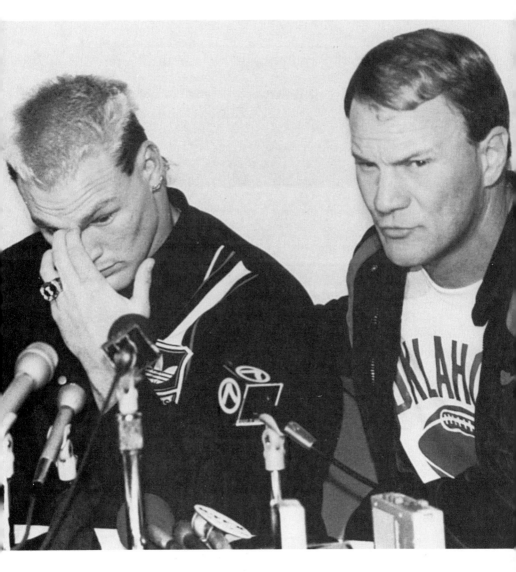

*Brian Bosworth (left) and coach Barry
Switzer face the press in 1986. Bosworth
admitted that he had taken steroids prescribed
by a doctor for injuries. He was banned
from playing in the 1987 Orange Bowl game.*

roids is also a profitable business. They want a share of the estimated $100 million a year that is spent on illegal steroids.

How Did Steroids Become So Popular?

The use of chemicals to improve athletic performance became a public issue in the Cold War era of the 1950s, when the Soviets made it clear they would do anything necessary to defeat Western athletes in Olympic contests of strength such as weight lifting. Soviet sports officials believed that synthesized hormones might provide the quick fix they needed to surpass their American rivals.

Earlier, steroids may have been used during the Second World War when Hitler's troops were given the substance to increase aggression, according to journalist Barry Cronin. Medical researcher L. T. Samuels and his associates reported that these substances were used in the 1930s to increase strength in aged men and to assist individuals with underdeveloped gonads. Researcher George L. White has noted that androgens were used in the 1940s to help emaciated prisoners of war gain weight.

By the 1950s, steroids were seen as wonder drugs that could fatten cattle quickly and were also thought to be a long-awaited cure for cancer. Since steroids were given to sick and malnourished people to make them better and bigger, the Soviets may have believed that there could be little harm in asking—or ordering—their male and female athletes to take straight testosterone as part of the conditioning process to prepare for the 1956 Olympic Games.

The United States won all the major weight-lifting and wrestling events, thanks to perhaps superior coaching and training techniques, and perhaps to negative steroid side-effects. However, it was clear that the Soviet

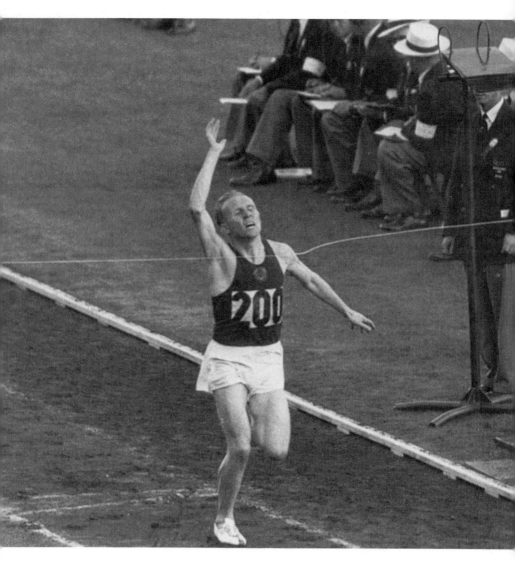

Russia's champion distance runner,
Vladimir Kuts, breasts the tape to win the
1956 Olympic 10,000-meter run in Melbourne,
Australia. Kuts broke the Olympic record
with a 28-minute, 45.6-second time.

Union and its satellite countries would be a formidable threat in future Olympic competitions.

"People used to question all the time [during the Olympics] why the East Germans were kept totally segregated and why their women all had very big voices and five o'clock shadows," said British Olympic swimmer Sharron Davies.[17] In time, these first Soviet competitors paid a heavy price for achieving better performances through chemicals. A few Russian male athletes became unable to urinate without using catheter tubes—an unusual condition in young men. By 1988, *Omni* magazine was able to document a high death rate among Soviet athletes, although it could only conjecture that steroid use might have killed them since the Russians shared no autopsy findings with the international press or Olympic authorities.[18]

Steroids in the
United States

During the late 1950s, few self-respecting American citizens wanted to play second fiddle to the Soviets, whether in the space race or a footrace. The United States had long dominated the Olympics because of its training and nutritional knowledge, but now it began to look as though the Soviets might gain an edge through chemical help. Consequently, the American doctor John B. Ziegler decided to investigate the possible athletic benefits of administering male-hormone compounds to athletes.[19]

Dr. Ziegler allied himself with a drug company named Ciba Pharmaceutical to give study subjects what he considered low dosages (5 mg) of testosterone extract. So safe did he consider this dosage that he administered it to himself to observe its effect.

From this cautious first step, it wasn't long before victory-conscious U.S. athletes were indulging themselves by taking tremendous dosages of steroids that re-

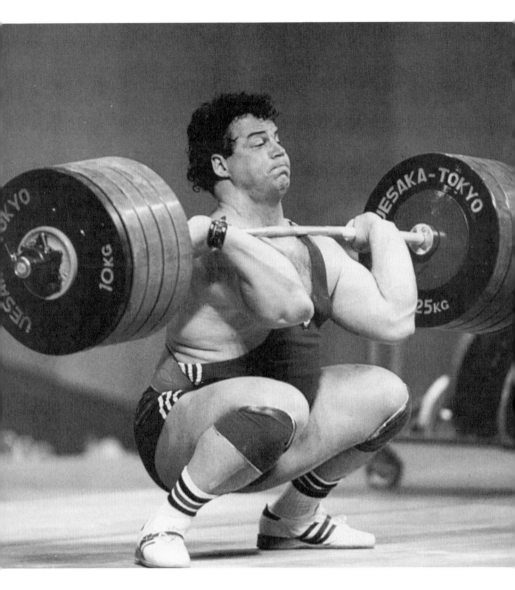

Russian weight lifter, Aleksandr Kourlovich, won the gold medal in the over-242-pound weight lifting event in the 1988 Olympics.

sulted in some severe physical problems. Shocked by the Frankenstein's monster he had built and unleashed, Dr. Ziegler discontinued his experimentation. But even without him, anabolic steroids were here to stay.

Athletes everywhere were convinced that hormones could give them what nature hadn't. "Drug use is like insider-trading scandals, scientists falsifying research, cheating by coaches," said Dr. Charles Yesalis. "They demonstrate that, to many people, the ends justify the means."[20]

According to veteran hurdler Edwin Moses, a non-user of steroids, by the 1980 Moscow Olympics things had deteriorated to a point where the governing bodies of many nations "were cutting deals" with one another. "A Western country would tell an East-bloc country, for example, that if they looked the other way while the Westerners rescinded the lifetime suspension of athlete A, then the East-bloc nation could reduce athlete B's ban from life to eighteen months," charged Moses.[21]

Recent evidence indicates that steroids are no longer tolerated, however, by Communist-bloc countries. In 1989 the United States and the Soviet Union signed a mutual drug-testing pact. One Moscow report acknowledged that authorities had punished 290 Soviet athletes for steroid use prior to the 1988 Olympic Games.[22]

The growing consensus, therefore, is that steroids are like many other quick-fix solutions in life. They may yield some early gains and victories, but they create real-life situations like the one that faced the legendary Faust, who sold his soul to the devil for a price. That devil may come calling later to extract a payment.

"Steroids can make you strong and beautiful," concluded another writer. "But if your body is polluted, the beauty is only skin deep."[23]

2
STEROIDS AS ILLICIT DRUGS

The Steroid Marketplace

Although steroids are drugs, many athletes rationalize taking them and convince themselves that they have nothing in common with users of street drugs like crack, cocaine, and PCP. But some athletes and fitness-minded men and women are like junkies in one respect. They are willing to break any law and go to any expense or trouble necessary to get the drug they think can help them.

Like the crack-cocaine addict who travels from crack house to crack house to get his or her needs satisfied, so, too, do athletes and fitness freaks search for suppliers of steroids and other size-enhancing drugs. There is no question that the steroid market rewards traffickers with large fortunes, an estimated $100 million in 1988 alone, according to federal authorities. Many owners and managers of fitness centers have made huge, untaxed profits by selling illicit steroids to their consumers, either directly or through intermediaries.

Dr. Michael Nelson, chairman of the American

31

Academy of Pediatrics Committee on Sports Medicine, estimates that an eight-week cycle of black-market steroids costs from $60 to $100—and that much of what is sold is of poor quality even when labeled with the names of legitimately manufactured drugs (when prescribed by a physician for proper purposes).[1]

Part of these profits (as high as 20 percent, claims one source) is made by unscrupulous physicians who provide steroids to athletes because they are greedy for high, quick profits or because they've rationalized that the athletes are going to buy steroids illegally, anyway, if the doctors don't provide them. Steroids sold by those physicians cost considerably more than black-market drugs, notes Dr. Nelson. In addition, many athletes think—like former Steeler Steve Courson, whose future now hinges on his ability to find a heart donor—that if a little helps, more ought to be even better. Therefore, many steroid users take doses that could put muscles on a half-dozen athletes—or steers, for that matter. The variety and amounts of steroids and drugs taken by athletes in training are simply horrifying.

One comprehensive study of female athletes who are steroid users demonstrated that they have the same mind-set as that of the many male athletes who use steroids. There is no limit to the amount of drugs that some women will take in order to win in their track-and-field events. The study was conducted by a physician named Richard H. Strauss, M.D.

The heaviest anabolic steroid user among ten women who trained with weights took daily oral doses of stanozolol (12 mg), oxandrolone (10 mg), and mesterolone (50 mg) for a ten-week cycle. In addition, during the last six weeks she injected 50 mg of a veterinary form of stanozolol twice a week, and in the final four weeks of the cycle, she injected 30 mg of methenolone acetate twice a week. These go whoppingly beyond manufacturers' recommendations—even if they weren't being taken in potentially dangerous combinations.

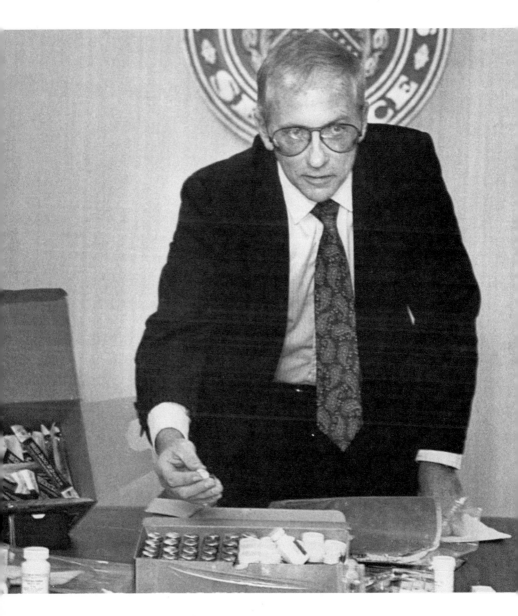

Patrick O'Brien, U.S. Special Agent in charge of U.S. Customs, at a press conference in May 1987 with steroids seized as part of a nationwide sweep of counterfeit steroids.

The amount of drugs all ten women used as a matter of course in training and competition staggers the imagination. It is also an indication of a mind-set that rationalizes, "Well, I'm already taking this huge storehouse of drugs anyway, so what's a few doses more?"

Here is the list the ten women gave Dr. Strauss and his research team of all the drugs they took for one reason or another (known brand names in parentheses):

- *Oral anabolic steroids:* mesterolone (Proviron), methandrostenolone (Dianabol—still known by this name on the black market even though the legitimate drug company that patented it has discontinued it), methenolone acetate (Primobolan), methyltestosterone, oxandrolone (Anavar), stanozolol (Winstrol).

- *Injectable anabolic steroids:* methandrostenolone (Dianabol in injectable form), methenolone enanthate, nandrolone decanoate (Deca-Durabolin), stenbolone acetate (Anatrofin), testosterone cypionate, mixture of testosterone esters (Sustanon 250).

- *Injectable anabolic steroids intended for veterinary use:* boldenone undecylenate (Equipoise), stanozolol (Winstrol-V).

- *Growth hormone*: somatotrophin (human growth hormone), rhesus growth hormone (unknown composition black-market drug).

- *Analgesic/anti-inflammatory agents:* acetaminophen and codeine (Tylenol with codeine), aspirin, benoxaprofen (Oraflex), naproxen (Naprosyn), oxycodone hydrochloride and aspirin (Percodan), phenybutazone (Butazolidin), piroxicam (Feldene).

- *Miscellaneous substances:* adrenalin (epinephrine); lanolin, menthol, methyl salicylate (Ben-Gay); caffeine pills, calcium, cholinine and inositol, dimethyl sulfoxide, electrolyte solution taken intravenously, Lasix (furosemide), levodopa, lidocaine (Xylocaine), potassium, suntan pills, thyroglobulin, vitamins of all types.[2]

This incredibly high number of drugs routinely taken by athletes helps explain why the fear most people have of taking drugs doesn't affect steroid users. "Coaches say, 'Hey, steroids are no good for you,' " said Steve Courson. "Well, how good is taking a painkiller in the ankle or the knee? The whole thing is hypocritical."[3]

Even more at risk are steroid users who do not try to balance their drug use by proper nutrition and a high-intensity strength program. According to Michael A. Nelson, M.D., these users will show few gains, and will also incur "tissue breakdown and loss of strength"—not to mention the same horrific side effects that threaten more knowledgeable steroid users. Steroids are useless for weight and strength gains unless used in conjunction with a significant training program.

Some athletes are desperate enough to inject themselves with steroids intended for veterinary use only. One of the most common veterinary steroids is the product known as boldenone undecyclenate, sold under the brand name Equipoise.[4]

Another common black-market substitute for expensive human growth hormone is called "rhesus growth hormone." Researchers are uncertain what the substance actually is made of, but rarely (and probably never) does it come from rhesus monkeys. They also doubt that it contains any growth hormone.[5]

Other Banned
Substances
Allegations made in June 1989 by Dr. Robert Kerr, a San Gabriel, California, physician and onetime proponent of

steroid use, indicated that steroids are not the only substance that athletes take to achieve an unfair advantage. *USA Today* published his charges that some Olympic-strength athletes sometimes combined strychnine and nerve gas with caffeine and barbiturates "to stimulate the central nervous system." He also stated that they took drugs known as neurotransmitters, which similarly stimulate the central nervous system.[6]

Moreover, according to Dr. Kerr, athletes from foreign nations willingly subjected their bodies to indignities to gain an unfair edge. He theorized that the Soviet-bloc nations boycotted the 1984 Olympic Games in Los Angeles—not for political reasons, but because they feared a sophisticated drug-testing system might expose their use of steroids and other illegal substances.

In the 1988 Games, he said, swimmers from the USSR "were injected with about 1½ quarts of air or gas in the rectum and colon to achieve better flotation."[7] Mexican race walkers—participants in an event that hardly rewards participants with either fame or fortune—injected themselves with pyruvate-dehydrogenase, charged Kerr, because this substance enhanced endurance.

Kerr's charges touched only the tip of the iceberg. Many archers, fencers, and marksmen use substances called beta blockers to slow their heart rates and steady their hands or trigger fingers.[8]

Diuretics are commonly used to help wrestlers and boxers make their weight classes. So is synthetic growth hormone, a drug with anabolic properties that, if taken in large doses (a commonplace practice) may cause enlargement of the heart, liver, and other organs.[9]

Archery competitor
Dave Hale in the
1988 Olympics.

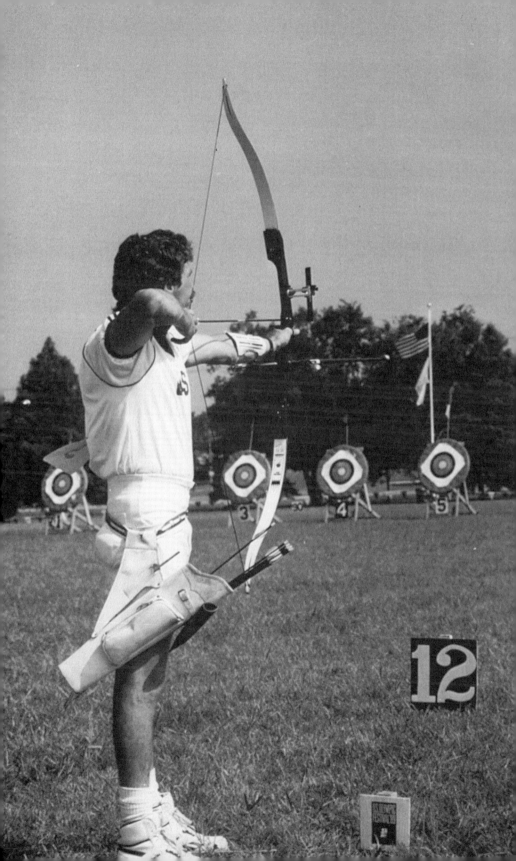

Some Athletes
Peddle Steroids

The network of steroid sellers is a chummy, close-knit one. "We can do a bust on one coast and within hours it is known everywhere in the country," one federal investigator told the *New York Times* reporters Peter Alfano and Michael Janofsky.[10]

In addition, one of the most appalling aspects of the black-market steroid trade is that many people who should be role models for youth are selling potentially harmful drugs. One of the most publicized arrests in the United States involved famous weight lifter Kotcha Doonkeen, a resident of Oklahoma City, Oklahoma, who was caught by U.S. Customs agents and charged with smuggling and delivering unprescribed anabolic steroids into another state.

In March 1989, a onetime Mr. Universe who boasted that his powerful physique came from "natural training" methods was busted on steroids-trafficking charges while in Ohio attending the Arnold Schwarzenegger Classic bodybuilding contest—an event honoring the actor, who says he built his remarkable body naturally.

The 1987 Mr. Universe, Luis I. Batista Freitas, was arrested along with his mother and an alleged accomplice by the U.S. Customs Service on charges of conspiracy and possession of anabolic steroids with intent to distribute. The arrest embarrassed members of the International Federation of Body Builders (IFBB) because their organization, of which Freitas was a member, has long taken an antisteroid stance.

Brazilian Luis Freitas
posing after winning
the heavyweight 1987
World Amateur Bodybuilding
Championship in Madrid.

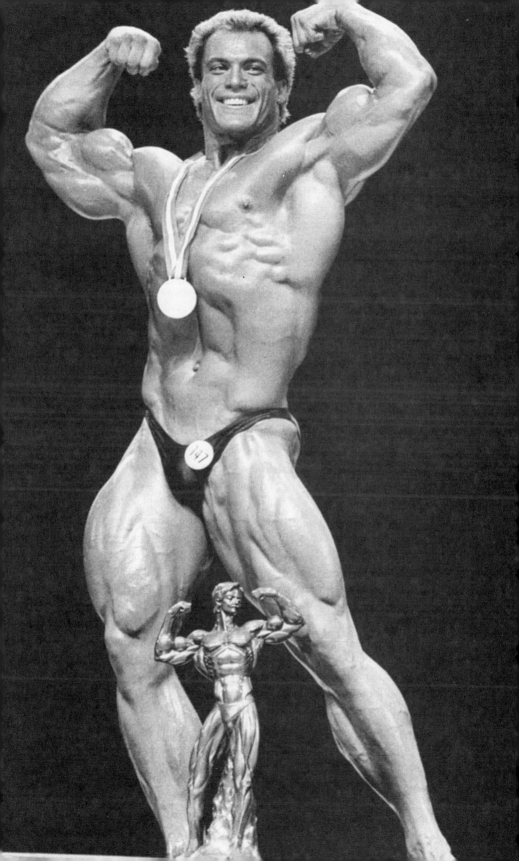

"We're very, very upset at what has happened, because we're trying to combat drugs not only in our sport, but in all sports," IFBB spokesman Harris Kegan told the Associated Press. "We've had a drug-testing program in place for years."[11]

Moreover, what is the parent of a college-bound athlete to think of admissions by three former University of South Carolina football coaches that they distributed steroids to their players?

"I had a sacred trust," Coach Jim Washburn told U.S. District Court judge G. Ross Anderson before the magistrate sentenced him and two colleagues to three months in a halfway house in lieu of prison cells. "I violated that."

Another major source of steroids for athletes over the years has been companies, many of them Mexican based, that offer black-market anabolic steroids by mail. Using leaflets and flyers that they send as "junk mail" at low postal rates, they offer muscle-building aids to anyone interested by way of the U.S. Postal Service, or various commercial delivery services. Both the House and Senate recently passed legislation prohibiting the sale of mail-order steroids. Fines and prison sentences are meted out to convicted violators. Nonetheless, the lure of easy profits keeps illegal laboratories in business.

Why do law enforcement experts feel that illegal steroid distribution should be prosecuted as a major crime? Mainly, they say, because black-market sellers may think twice about selling banned drugs if they know a felony charge may result.

Many sports-medicine experts are convinced that simply educating athletes about the dangers of steroids is not enough to deter them. "You can educate the athlete as much as possible, but until you add a punitive arm to this program, you don't get their attention," said U.S. Olympic Committee team physician Dr. Roy T. Bergman.[12]

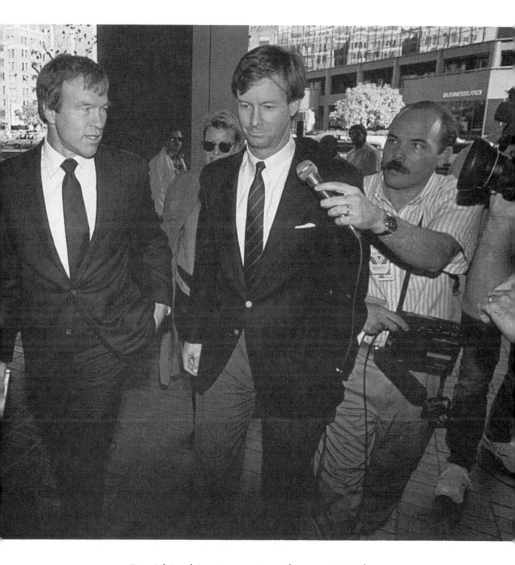

David Jenkins (center), a former British Olympian, accused of masterminding an international steroid smuggling ring out of Tijuana, Mexico, on his way into U.S. District Court in 1987. Jenkins pleaded guilty to 4 of the original 110 counts.

"Educating our students isn't enough," added Dr. Edward Wojtys, a member of NCAA drug-testing teams. "Athletes have shown us that they will do just about whatever they have to just to win or gain a competitive edge."[13]

The federal penalties for steroid trafficking are severe. The Omnibus Anti-Substance Abuse Act of 1988 shored up penalties for peddling steroids. Trafficking, which had been a misdemeanor, became a felony punishable by three years in prison and a $25,000 fine. The penalties are doubled if the customer is a minor.

Even doctors no longer can prescribe steroids if a patient intends to use the drug for athletic gains.

Laws against steroid use or distribution vary from state to state. In Indiana, for example, where I live, using or distributing anabolic steroids is a felony, a major crime. Just as laws vary from state to state, so does the degree of vigor with which state law enforcement officials pursue convictions of steroid traffickers. Some states, including Indiana, have had only a handful of arrests, perhaps reflecting a lack of vigorous pursuit by law enforcement officials more than any paucity of users. A former University of Indiana football player told me, for example, that a few players on his team were experimenting with steroids even ten years ago, when Lee Corso was coaching. But California, the traditional mecca for fitness freaks, has had many steroid busts. A single U.S. Attorney in the county of San Diego prosecuted 151 cases from 1985 to 1988.[14]

Profile of a Dealer

In the spring of 1986, while serving as adviser to the campus magazine at Ball State University in Muncie, Indiana, I assigned student writer Tim Walker (a weight lifter who achieved his muscular body naturally) to spend time with a local steroid peddler who agreed to talk as long as we referred to him in print as "Jake," a pseudonym. The dealer was a bodybuilder who gained his size from doses of the medicine he now sold to others. Walker said the man covered his massive torso with several shirts, as if "one is insufficient to cover him," and favored the briefest of shorts, which revealed the muscular definition of his legs.

Jake also was a student at Ball State and claimed to be making enough money from selling prescription drugs in a Central Indiana gym to finance his education in style. (Jake owned a membership in a second gym, where he worked out only, and where he refused to sell steroids.)

The dealer sold steroids intended for veterinary use as well as those most commonly used by humans, but refused to sell street drugs such as cocaine and marijuana, although he said he received many requests for both. He also refused to sell steroids to nonathletes and non-bodybuilders, although he admitted that he had received requests from people "who wanted to take them without even lifting"—for cosmetic reasons only.

The majority of his sales, he insisted, were by referral, and so he didn't feel as though he should be lumped with drug pushers. "I really don't feel bad about what I'm doing," he said. "People come to me for the 'roids; I don't go to them."

Later, however, he admitted that his conscience bothered him whenever a teenager requested steroids. "We would all be better off if they had never been invented," he said. "When I get out of school, I'm quitting this s——."

Significantly, writer Tim Walker observed Jake refusing to sell steroids to a fifteen-year-old boy who requested them during an interview held at a Muncie gym.

"Listen, lift hard for a year and eat like crazy," Jake advised the boy. "If you don't gain a lot of weight in that year, then hang up bodybuilding. Just don't rely on drugs."[15]

Steve Courson, even back in 1985, when he was devouring steroids in incredible quantities, advised young people to stay off steroids because the drugs do the most harm to maturing bodies. Courson, who went from 225 pounds to 260 in his sophomore year at that onetime hotbed of steroid use, the University of South Carolina, said, "I never recommend steroids to high school kids. I tell them they're too young. I say, 'Wait until you get everything you can from your body, naturally.' "[16]

But Jake, the Indiana dealer, is small potatoes compared to larger syndicates of sellers whose profits dwarf those made at gyms and health clubs. Other large profits are made by pharmacists who illegally sell—often in bulk—steroids such as Anadrol-50 (used by prescription by bone marrow patients) to athletes and bodybuilders they believe will not report them. Because steroids are less publicized and considered less dangerous than hard street drugs, many sellers work with little fear of apprehension by law enforcement agencies.

When dealer Charles J. Radler of Pittsburgh was busted in 1984, it was estimated that he grossed $20,000 a week. In one nine-month period, he deposited $673,000 in four bank accounts.[17]

3
STEROIDS IN SPORTS

Everyone Does It
Or So "They" Say

Why do athletes take steroids? Why do coaches condone their use? The answer is simple. Contrary to the old
sports slogan that says, "Cheaters never win," the evidence shows that many superstars in sports ranging from
baseball to weight lifting gain a substantial, although
unfair, edge by indulging in illegal substances. In addition, although steroids have many negative health aspects, they are popular among athletes, who believe
there is little or no risk of death so long as they use
steroids in proper dosages.

U.S. Olympic Committee chief medical officer, Dr.
Robert Voy, says he has observed three different reac-
tions to steroid use in athletes: (1) no effect; (2) some
effect, but users get "sick"; (3) they "almost grow as you
sit in front of them."[1]

Enough athletes achieve substantial athletic gains
from steroids to make nonusers decide to try them. "I

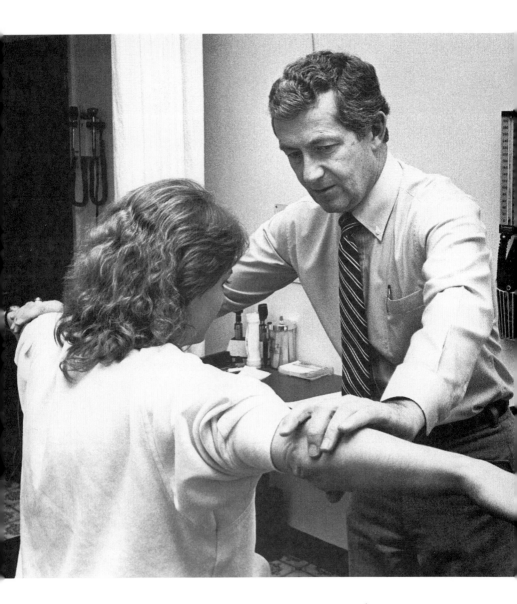

Dr. Robert Voy, manager of sports medicine
at the U.S. Olympic Training Center
in Colorado Springs, works with Jill
Stokesberry, an Olympic judo hopeful.

think it's got to the stage where everybody is doing it because it's the only way they can compete," swimmer Sharron Davies told the Associated Press. "I want to win desperately, and if I thought there would be no side effects and I wasn't going to be caught, then I would take them."[2]

Steve Courson still believes that he wasn't cheating when he took steroids regularly during his years in the NFL from 1977 to 1985. He calls it "maintaining parity" and says that those who never played the game can't understand the pressures on a player to take drugs to aid strength and size. "An ethics professor . . . never had to go head to head with a 295-pound armored warrior," said Courson. "I could not have stayed in the NFL without steroids—not on the line of scrimmage. I had 21-inch arms. I didn't get that big eating my Wheaties."[3]

Courson's former coach, Chuck Noll, has been known to chew out players who have talked about their steroid use. His position on the size he prefers his players to be is unequivocal. "We don't prefer small, quick, people," he once said. "We'd like to have big, quick people."

Is there any wonder that the NFL routinely now lists 40 players at 300 pounds or better on its preseason rosters?

When Brian Bosworth was caught taking steroids by the NCAA, he echoed the sentiments of many athletes, declaring that he'd done nothing wrong since he hadn't been taking so-called drugs. "I'll continue to fight against the abuse of drugs—recreational drugs that are destroying society," he told a press conference. "Steroids aren't destroying society."

What they (Boz and others) are destroying, however, is the integrity of the game and the fans' belief that on a given day it is the most talented team that will come out on top. "When two teams are nearly equal, the steroid team will win every time," complained former University of Michigan football coach Bo Schembechler, a man praised by his peers for his refusal to cheat.[4]

Unlike Schembechler, many coaches, school boards, boosters, and team owners have directly or indirectly contributed to steroid use by fostering a win-at-all-costs atmosphere. Nearly all use of steroids—particularly steroids injected in legs, stomach muscles, buttocks, and arms—is obvious to a trained coach. Yet few coaches want to *really* know that their team's winning chemistry is actually winning through chemistry.

There is no question that despite their denials some coaches put pressure on their athletes to take steroids. Even at the high school level, where damage to steroid-using adolescents is estimated to be the greatest, a few unscrupulous coaches either look the other way to avoid seeing steroid abuse or actually condone or even recommend their use by athletes. "To say every coach wants to rid his program of steroids is a little naive," admits Skip Morris, executive director of the national High School Athletic Coaches Association.[5] Particularly when the coach himself is a current or former steroid user!

Moreover, coaches are reluctant to drop talented steroid users from their squad, let alone report drug abuse to higher authorities. The *New York Times* reported an instance in which a college football coach tried to "hide" a steroid user during a drug test and, when unsuccessful, blasted the testing doctor for trying to sabotage his team's success.

Other coaches, aware that their reputations and jobs depend on winning games, aren't particular about whom they play. Jim Bouton, the former New York Yankee pitcher, once said—not entirely in jest—that managers would play a mass murderer like Charles Manson if they thought he could hit .300.

Perhaps Ben Johnson is the best example of an athlete led astray by poor advice, according to the sprinter's attorney, Ed Futerman. The attorney told *USA Today* that Johnson might not have understood the consequences of taking steroids. He intimated that Johnson's coach, Charlie Francis, was interested more in winning than in his player's physical well-being when he introduced Johnson to steroids at the age of nineteen.[6]

Certainly Charlie Francis forever damaged his own credibility when he denied responsibility for giving Johnson steroids, claiming at the Olympics that a spiked drink was given the sprinter. When an investigation took place, Francis changed his tune, documenting prolonged use of steroids by Johnson since 1981.

Thankfully, however, there are many coaches with strong ethical beliefs who are unwilling to risk their athletes' lives for a few more percentage points in the win column.

Boston College head football coach Jack Bicknell said he believes that coaches who use such shortcuts to success as steroids or engaging in recruiting violations are doing a disservice to their players. "Sure, there's pressure to win and to put people in the stands," Bicknell told United Press International. "But you can't let the pressure get to you. When working with kids, you can't let them believe that the easy way will help them to succeed."[7]

However, it would be naive of coaches and educators to think that athletes won't grab an edge to move ahead of the competition—regardless of whether that edge is real or imagined. Gladiators in Greco-Roman times tried to get a similar edge by eating the hearts of valiant opponents they had vanquished and the meat of powerful or fast-running animals.[8]

Maintaining Parity

When the Russians began using steroids in 1954, it wasn't long before the United States followed. And when steroids were shown to work for power lifters, discus throwers, and shot putters, it wasn't long before wrestlers, swimmers, football players, and track athletes were using them as well. Now there is scarcely a sport in the world that doesn't have one or more athletes trying to get ahead through chemicals. Athletes (and others) have a tendency to perform better if they think they're taking some drug purported to work magic. Some athletes were given placebos but thought they were given anabolic steroids and showed remarkable gains in competition because they were psychologically motivated.[9]

Steroids have been forced on athletes in Soviet-bloc nations, according to one defector. Christine Knacke, an East German swimmer who broke the one-minute barrier for the 100-meter butterfly, said, "I was doped, but not at my own will."[10]

In the United States, several track stars have charged that their coaches used subtle pressure and threats to get them to use steroids. No one, however, has said that he or she was forced directly to use chemicals while competing.

Because athletes who use anabolic steroids gain an unfair advantage over their peers, many in the world of college athletics believe penalties should be severe. Nonusers are angered by the thought of how many world records have been set while athletes were taking performance-enhancing drugs. Both Carl Lewis and Mary Decker Slaney, who say they are nonusers, claim that the majority of Olympic competitors take anabolic steroids.

"The penalties need to be stronger," University of Notre Dame athletic trainer Jim Russ told the [Hammond] *Times*. "If a kid tests positive for steroid usage, maybe he should be done for a year, or even a career."[11]

Without question, the number of track-and-field athletes who use steroids to enhance performance is alarmingly high. In track and field, only long-distance running events are relatively free of steroid users, and this is

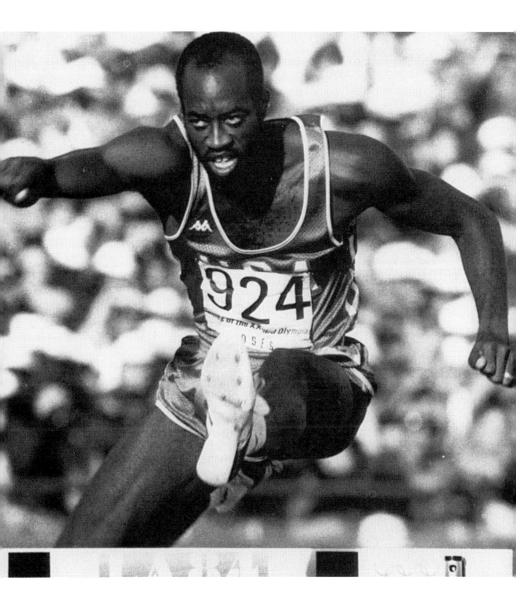

Edwin Moses, shown here running the 400-meter hurdles event in the 1984 Olympics, has been an outspoken critic of steroid use.

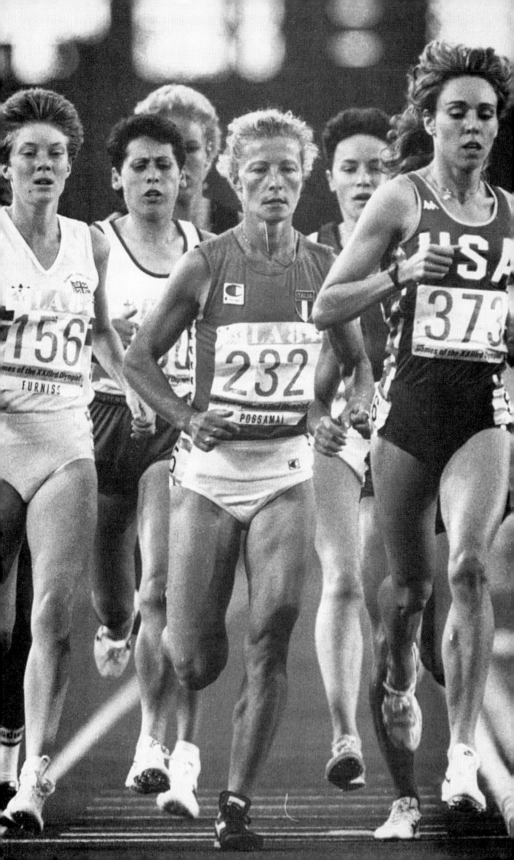

because drugs are thought not to help in those events. A doctor who admitted supplying steroids to thousands of athletes for nearly twenty years (until he perceived the dangers to be enough to convince him to discontinue the practice in 1984) estimated that 90 percent of all Olympic athletes have used one banned drug or another. Dr. Robert Kerr admitted that he prescribed steroids to "about twenty" Olympians at the 1984 Olympics.[12]

The Case That
Shook the World

Ben Johnson's admission that he used steroids to win in the 1988 Olympic Games in Seoul, South Korea, created an international furor. The general public had been aware of steroid abuse for years. But the public somehow accepted the image of beefy football linemen and Olympic shot putters—particularly if they were from the Soviet Union—taking the drug. In fact, hardly any reporters raised eyebrows in Seoul when *U.S. News & World Report* noted that IOC vice-president Richard Pound thought that weight lifting was so fraught with cheaters that it should no longer be an Olympic sport.

What caused an uproar was the confirmation,

Mary Decker Slaney (373) leads the pack on her way to winning the first heat of the 3,000-meter race in the 1984 Olympic Games. Following her are Agnese Possamai of Italy (232) and Jane Furniss (156) of Great Britain.

seventy-two hours after the running of the 100-meter sprint, that the world's fastest human had used steroids to take precious microseconds off his time. Suddenly, in the public's perception, all track-and-field athletes were tainted. For several months stars such as Florence Griffith Joyner and her sister-in-law, Jackie Joyner-Kersee, could not appear in public without a reporter demanding if they, too, were taking performance-enhancing drugs—the controversy fueled by remarks on their integrity by Carl Lewis and other athletes.

Griffith Joyner, in fact, said she would sue Carl Lewis or any other person who linked her name with steroids. A sad aspect of the whole steroid controversy has been that many successful athletes who have achieved success without chemicals have been branded drug users by their competitors and the general public. "I'm sick and tired of all the innuendo," Griffith Joyner told David Leon Moore of *USA Today*. "It's not right and it's not fair."[13]

But after the Ben Johnson incident, an official inquiry into substance abuse ordered by Prime Minister Brian Mulroney of Canada revealed that an alarming number of international track-and-field superstars have, indeed, cheated their way to fame and sometimes fortune.

The Commission of Inquiry into the Use of Drugs and Banned Practices Intended to Increase Athletic Performance grilled Ben Johnson himself and learned that the twenty-seven-year-old runner was a longtime user of

Florence Griffith Joyner,
1988 U.S. Olympic winner
of three gold and
one silver medal in
track and field.

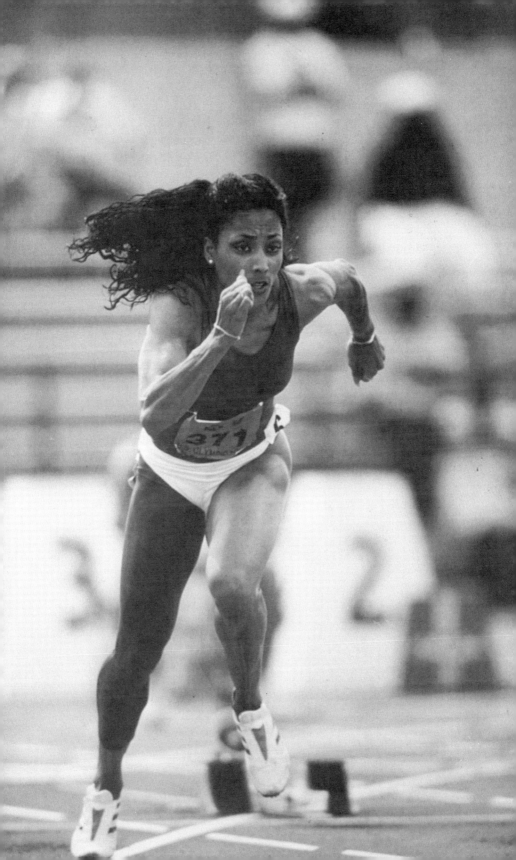

anabolic steroids, pure testosterone, and human growth hormone. As early as 1981, the sprinter said, he began taking stanozolol and other steroids. He was one of twelve athletes trained by Charlie Francis who took banned substances, according to testimony given at the hearing.

The coach justified his condoning of drugs by saying he felt the majority of international competitors took them and that he wanted his athlete to remain competitive.[14]

Team Sanctions:
The Wave of the Future

Heretofore, when an athlete has tested positive for steroids, he or she has accepted the shame and the blame. In the future, however, says NCAA executive director Richard D. Schultz, there also may be sanctions against college teams that have violators on the roster. "There are some concerns . . . whether the whole team should be penalized by the indiscretions of the individual," Schultz told the *Myrtle Beach* [South Carolina] *Sun.*[15]

If the NCAA Executive Committee feels that teams should suffer sanctions for knowingly or unknowingly allowing illegal drug users to compete, it has the option of establishing legislation that would result in penalties. The NCAA began random, year-round testing of college football players for performance-enhancing drugs in 1990.

Some college coaches, however, feel that the NCAA is putting them in the law enforcement business. Phillip P. "Sparky" Woods—head football coach of the University of South Carolina, which suffered a steroid scandal under Joe Morrison, his predecessor—argued that coaches should not be held responsible for the irresponsible actions of their players as long as they do everything possible to discourage the use of steroids. "I do not think somebody ought to persecute me because one of those hundred-and-something, twenty-year-old [players] messes up," said Woods.[16] It should also be noted that a University of South Carolina internal study in 1990 revealed that in at least one instance a Gamecock coach had suggested that a player should consider taking steroids.

His contention is an interesting one. How much blame should be put squarely on the backs of the athletes? How much should be placed on parents, particularly if the athlete is under eighteen?

College and Professional Football: Repeat Offenders

Although the case of Olympic sprinter Ben Johnson was the most publicized, one expert cautioned against condemning all runners because of Johnson's transgressions. "We're kind of condemning runners," said Dr. Robert Kerr, former prescriber of steroids. "Yet they probably take fewer drugs overall than [do athletes in] many, many other sports."[17]

The sport in which the temptation is greatest because of the need for sheer brute strength is football. Because of the fired-up mentality of a steroid user, coaches tended, for years, to see users as assets instead of liabilities. Consequently, the NFL looked upon steroid offenders with much more benevolence than they did street drug users.

"It's wrong for the NFL to draw a distinction between cocaine, marijuana, and steroids," said Kim Wood, strength coach for the Cincinnati Bengals. "Steroids are just as dangerous to the user, maybe more dangerous. But look at it this way: If a coach has a guy who's screwed up on cocaine, he'll have trouble coaching the guy. On the other hand, if a player's juiced up on steroids, he'll play like he's fighting on Guadalcanal. He's not only not a problem, he's an asset to the team."[18]

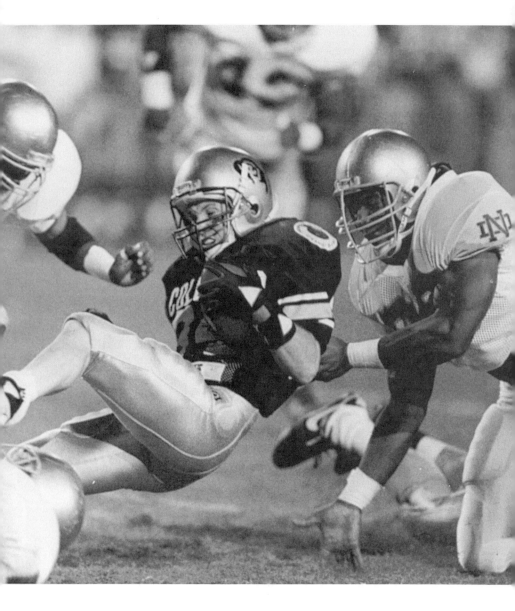

*Colorado's wide receiver Jeff Campbell (84)
goes down at the hands of Notre Dame
defenders in the 1990 Orange Bowl Classic.*

All-pro Atlanta Falcon guard Bill Fralic, a onetime steroid user who now denounces the drugs, told a U.S. Senate panel that their use by football players was part of a predictable bad cycle. "High school players think they need steroids to win a college scholarship. College players do steroids so they can improve their chances at playing in the pros and getting a lucrative contract. NFL players use steroids to keep their jobs because there are few guaranteed contracts in our league."

Fralic's conclusion? "The system rewards you for being a good football player, no matter what the means are to the end."[19]

Perhaps the most damning conclusion about the governing bodies in sport was made by top miler Steve Scott. "The National Football League and NCAA talk a mean story," scoffed Scott. "But when it comes down to 'Are [they] helping the youth of America stay healthy?' the answer is no."[20]

4

STEROIDS IN SOCIETY

4

A Muscle Mentality

Although pinpointing an exact figure is impossible because steroid use is shrouded in secrecy, medical researchers believe that between 1 and 3 million youths and adults have taken anabolic steroids in one form or another specifically to enhance their looks or athletic performances. Unless the mentality that encourages short-term gains at long-term expense is changed, indications are that many more millions of people will try steroids over the next few years.

Why?

Researcher Charles E. Yesalis of the Pennsylvania State University Department of Health and Human Development blamed it on our social environment. "Large segments of society accept the use of drugs," he wrote in a syndicated column that appeared in the *New York Times.* "We use drugs to lose weight, to stop pain, to keep awake, to put us to sleep and to create feelings of pleasure. We pop a lot of pills and we have come to expect from modern technology—drugs included—faster and better results and effects.

"We are also a highly competitive society where a win-at-any-cost philosophy prevails. Quite simply, also-rans, regardless of their effort, are rewarded disproportionately, if at all."[1]

A Chicago steroid dealer, who was a self-described "twerp" in high school, explained the demand for his product in lay terms. "It makes you feel like you can be anything you wanna be," said the twenty-four-year-old dealer who claimed to make $1,000 a week. "There's only one guy in 100,000 who's a natural athlete, and that's why people want steroids."[2]

Professor Yesalis said that cheating athletes and law-breaking fitness freaks are just another symptom of a bruised society that also experiences Wall Street insider-trading scandals, falsified research by scientists, and industrial spying. "If a potentially harmful drug were available that would significantly increase the productivity of college professors, we might well see a level of use of the drug in academia similar to that of steroids in sports," he wrote.[3]

Dr. Robert Waite, a former Idaho State University professor and now a U.S. Justice Department researcher, agreed with Yesalis's theory. "When I was a skinny kid in high school I wanted nothing more than to play hockey," he told me. "I'm glad steroids weren't popular when I was growing up—I'm sure I would have taken them."

Moreover, people today want immediate gratification and immediate results. The old-fashioned body-building methods don't work fast enough for those willing to risk their health in exchange for powerful builds in three to six months. "Before, the ninety-seven-pound weakling on the beach turned to weight lifting," a Florida physician told *Time*. "Now he turns to steroids."[4]

One 5-foot-6-inch, 115-pound, seventeen-year-old from Boston agreed, saying he recently began taking steroids orally to increase his size. "I'm sick of being small," he said. "I want to be bigger."[5]

Wealthy students in the suburbs and the poor of inner-city ghettos are willing to spend hard cash for a drug that gives the user a high only when he or she looks in the mirror. One dealer who had paid $2,000 for 200 bottles of Dianabol (a one-month supply of pills) resold them for $35 a bottle. Injectable forms of anabolic steroids command a much higher price. Many suppliers simply get their steroids from one of several Latin American countries, where they are sold in drugstores over the counter.[6]

The Dianabol dealer admits selling to high school students but suffers pangs of conscience. "It started to bother me when it got into the high schools because the kids don't know what they're doing," he said. "They won't grow as tall because it . . . stunts your growth."[7]

Depression and Suicide

Another problem for young people who take steroids is that they can lead to severe depression when the user decides to stop. "If you're on steroids at high doses, it can be bad to kick them without professional help," said Dr. Kirk Brower of the University of Michigan psychiatry department. "Deep depression is one of the withdrawal symptoms of getting off steroids."[8]

Several youths have committed suicide while on steroids or trying to come off them. A Chicago youth, for example, was secretly taking steroids while seeing several doctors for treatment of depression. Unaware that he was a steroid user, the doctors failed to make the proper diagnosis. He hanged himself in his closet with a favorite tie.[9]

Another problem with injecting steroids is that users frequently share needles while injecting, leaving themselves open to all sorts of diseases, from hepatitis to AIDS. In July 1989, for example, a bodybuilder told a U.S. Olympic Committee physician, Dr. Michael Scott, that he had gotten AIDS from sharing a needle with an infected fellow lifter while injecting steroids.[10]

An International
Problem

Surprising admissions by Vasily Gromyko, deputy chairman of the Soviet State Committee for Physical Culture and Sports, have shown that steroids are also regarded as a societal problem in the Soviet Union—and not only among athletes. "Mr. Sylvester Stallone and Mr. Arnold Schwarzenegger are very popular in our country," said Gromyko. "This is because of their strong builds." He concluded that Soviet drug problems were not confined to athletes, but that adolescents were also likely to use steroids.[11]

The vast majority of steroid users are young men. Women may take the drug to enhance athletic performance or to acquire a muscular build, but few young women are attracted to taking steroids.

Syndicated columnist Patricia McLaughlin finds it ironic that young men wishing to look better will take steroids that can make them, in the long run, only less attractive to the opposite sex. "Scrawny teenagers take the drug to be big and powerful, and it fuses their long bones so they stop growing," scoffs McLaughlin, who says she wonders where are the brains of users who don't know the difference between aspirin and Dianabol. "Guys take steroids to be macho and end up with shriveled gonads."[12]

Some Revealing
Surveys

Surveys regarding use of illegal performance-enhancing drugs have turned up data that have distressed the general public. The use of such substances has proved to be far more widespread than was thought possible. A national study by the American Medical Association indicated that 6.6 percent of male high school seniors have had or continue to have some involvement with anabolic steroids. Moreover, six out of every ten seniors say they purchase black-market drugs.[13]

"The problem is of sufficient magnitude that it would be inappropriate for any high school administration or coach to assume their school is not at risk," concluded Charles E. Yesalis.[14]

The 1987 study conducted by Yesalis at Pennsylvania State University found that as many as half a million teenage males have used steroids. Moreover, nearly 27 percent (26.7 percent) of steroid users they questioned admitted they took the substance only to enhance their looks, not for athletic gain.

"I didn't have any idea it would be this high," assistant professor W. E. Buckley of Penn State told the Associated Press. "It's the new-age, body beautiful, fitness people out there as well [as athletes] who are using anabolic steroids."[15]

A 1987 study performed by the University of Arkansas turned up similar information but also demonstrated that teenagers who used steroids were ill informed about the possible long-term ill effects of such use. The Arkansas researchers interviewed 853 adolescent men at six high schools and found that 10 percent had used or were using steroids.

According to Steve Tally of *Men's Fitness* magazine, nearly 20 percent of all steroid users wrongly believed the drugs would enhance their aerobic performance. Steroids may increase strength and even speed, but not aerobic performance. In addition, 12 percent took them because they mistakenly thought steroids could make them taller, and nearly 33 percent were unaware the drugs could actually stunt growth. Even more disturbing,

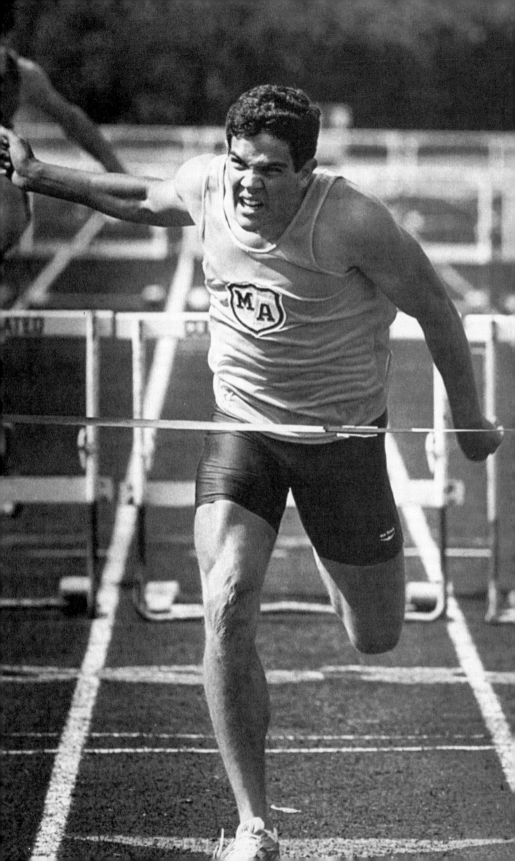

nearly four out of ten students said they had no idea steroids might cause liver damage.

Other revealing aspects of the Arkansas survey were the following:

Eighty-four percent of the users were athletes who wanted to gain an edge over the opposition.

Thirty-three percent thought steroids would improve their appearance.

Ten percent took steroids, as one respondent put it, "because, like, all of the dudes are doin' it."[16]

The New "Breakfast" of Wanna-Be Champions

In November 1988, Philip Halpern, a U.S. Attorney in San Diego, claimed that the steroid problem outside the athletic community is far more serious than previously thought. Halpern estimated that 90 percent of steroid sales are made to males who do not participate in competitive sports but are obsessed with their appearance. "The majority of steroids are consumed by individuals who are concerned by how they look—factory workers, lawyers, and firemen—and there is even a smaller market now in kids," said Halpern.[17]

Contrary to what authorities might expect, the average person on the street interested in steroids has not

A high school regional track meet winner pushing to win the hurdles event.

been deterred by the suspensions of prominent football players and Olympic athletes.

"The day after Ben Johnson tested positive for steroids and was stripped of his Olympic medal, hundreds of kids were calling their local gyms asking where they could get some Winstrol [an anabolic steroid]," said Dr. Bob Goldman of Chicago.[18]

5

POSSIBLE SIDE EFFECTS

From "Chemical Man" to Invalid

Following on the heels of a 1989 Canadian inquiry into the use of steroids by sprinter Ben Johnson and other top athletes came the announcement by a onetime steroid abuser that he needed a heart transplant. Steve Courson, was known as "the Chemical Man" to his fellow NFL pros because he built his giant body on a longtime diet of steroids.

The former NFL offensive lineman with Pittsburgh and Tampa Bay had admitted just four years earlier to *Sports Illustrated* that he was a steroid abuser. Now, reported *USA Today*, he was diagnosed with dilated cardiomyopathy—in lay terms, a worn-out heart—and he was a doomed man unless he obtained a heart transplant, something that had not yet occurred by December 1989.

Steve Courson, in 1989, was only thirty-three.

Like most steroid users who have suffered irreversible health problems, Courson can't say for sure that the

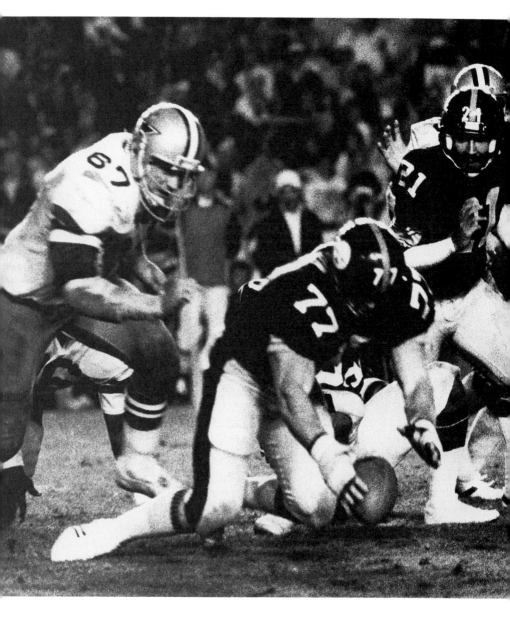

*Steve Courson (77) playing for
the Pittsburgh Steelers in 1979.*

drugs were responsible for putting his life in jeopardy. Then again, he can't say that they didn't. "That's the crux of the whole steroids problem," he said. "There is so much we just don't know yet."[1]

Steroid Research:
Behind the Times

Because steroid research has failed to keep up with steroid use, physicians are reluctant to condemn steroids outright. For one thing, so many doctors (and the prestigious American College of Sports Medicine) had doubted the effectiveness of steroids to improve strength and performance that they lost credibility with athletes and highly informed underground experts who witnessed results to the contrary. Thus, many athletes smirked when the president of the American College of Sports Medicine, Dr. Lyle Micheli, in 1989 said that "the potential health hazard [of steroids] is very frightening."[2] What these athletes want is overwhelming anecdotal evidence; that simply is not going to happen except in rare cases when athletes go public, as did Courson with his health problems.

Athletes also object because anabolic steroids, after all, have been approved by the Food and Drug Administration (FDA) for certain skin ailments and other maladies, although the FDA prohibits them from being used to enhance strength or athletic performance. (The FDA does acknowledge that steroids may do both, however.) Many doctors are reluctant to condemn a drug because it has some adverse side effects. Few, if any, drugs don't affect *someone* adversely.

Therefore, the team physician for the Cleveland Cavaliers, Dr. John A. Lombardo, cautions that it is wrong to equate steroids with such a deadly poison as cyanide, or clearly addictive "pleasure" drugs like crack, cocaine, or heroin. However, Dr. Lombardo feels there are risks with the drugs and refuses to prescribe them. The *New York*

Times has cited experts who compare the danger of using steroids with the danger of taking birth control pills. And yet no one has ever documented a woman taking a hundred times the prescribed dose for birth control pills to prevent pregnancy, as athletes have done with steroids to get fast and significant strength and size gains.[3]

Many physicians believe that there is a direct link between steroid use and serious health problems; they cite strong circumstantial evidence to condemn the drugs. Athletes, on the other hand, all know steroid users who have taken the drugs in large quantities for long periods of time without apparent ill effects. It may be years before valid studies are available.

A Bad Bargain
for Adolescents

All the evidence seems to indicate that steroids can be a bad bargain, particularly for those who abuse the drug and for adolescents whose bodies have not stopped growing. If you are one of the unlucky users, you must be willing to sacrifice your health in later years in exchange for a pumped-up body today. One joke making the rounds of gyms is that steroid users don't care if they die so long as they look good in the coffin.[4]

Interpreting
the Evidence

One reason that clinical evidence about effects of steroid use is so paltry is that researchers have found it both ethically and practically undesirable to conduct any sort of organized testing. Hence, studies have depended heavily on just a handful of surveys of steroid users. And Michael A. Nelson, chairman of the American Academy of Pediatric Medicine, stresses these were based on inaccurate reports. Dr. Nelson notes that athletes often won't admit to a researcher that they use steroids. On the other hand, a middle school student, hoping to impress and to be thought of as with it, may falsely tell a researcher that he or she uses steroids. Quite possibly, exact figures may never be available.

Investigators are also loath to attribute a death to steroid use when other factors are present. One five-year user of steroids dropped dead of a heart attack at twenty-seven. However, there may have been other factors involved. For example, the victim's father had died of a heart attack at thirty-two, and this could be seen as evidence of a predisposition toward heart disease.

Steve Courson—who believes that up to 3 million people in this country have tried steroids—is not the only steroid user to suffer horrendous effects. Here are some other cases that have drawn national attention.

In April 1988, *Newsweek* stated that the West German heptathlete Birgit Dressel "died of an immune-system breakdown that reportedly was brought on by steroid abuse."[5]

A Pennsylvania bodybuilder, Rocky Rauch, in 1989 blamed steroid use as the cause of his cancer.[6]

On January 10, 1989, the Ashtabula (Ohio) County coroner's office concluded "a contributing factor" in the death of a seventeen-year-old high school football player, Benji Ramirez, the previous October, was steroid use.

But "contributing to death," of course, is not the same as being "the cause of death." Until doctors and sports administrators can unequivocally say that steroids have caused a fatality, athletes and other fitness buffs undoubtedly will refuse to listen.

"If all of a sudden you had empirical data that said 137 American athletes died in the '76 Olympic games and anabolic steroids did it, you would have people sit

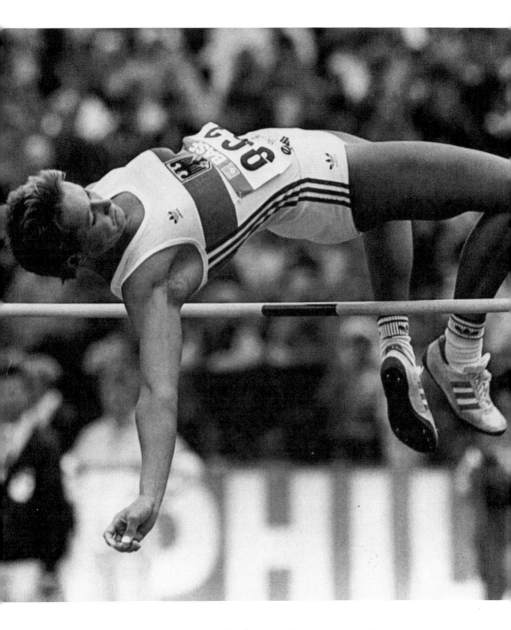

*Birgit Dressel of West Germany easily
clears the bar on her way to a jump of 1.92
meters in a women's heptathlon competition.*

up and take notice," former Olympic weight lifter Bruce Wilhelm, a U.S. Olympic Committee executive board member, told the *New York Times*. "But they have not been able to link one death to it."

Even if someday steroids are declared life threatening, many athletes and drug experts feel that people will continue to take them. "The Surgeon General says one in every six deaths is linked to cigarettes," said Courson. "And yet millions of people still smoke."[7]

What Are the Risks?

A study of the available research shows that there are some health hazards and some adverse results that a heavy steroid user can expect to encounter. In adolescent users, there is a strong risk of stunted growth because of a reduction in bone growth. All users can expect tendon and muscle pulls that take far longer than normal to heal. This happens because these muscles and tendons are handling bulk that nature never intended them to have, or because they have not yet become accustomed to handling that extra body mass.

"Eighty percent of the time when a big guy tears a muscle, steroids are probably the reason," said Howie Long of the Los Angeles Raiders, who charged in *Sports Illustrated* that 75 percent of offensive linemen use drugs. "You put 50 pounds of muscle on a player, and . . . something has to give. You're putting too much muscle fiber on a body not designed for it."[8]

As with any drug taken in excess, there may be an adverse reaction in blood pressure and the way bodily organs respond to the chemical. "My heart was going 160 beats per minute, and it scared the hell out of me," noted Steve Courson.[9] Anabolic steroids have been linked to high blood pressure and clogging of the arteries due to high cholesterol. Proponents of steroids shrug off such announcements, pointing out that other factors might have caused such symptoms.

What are the worst steroids to take, from a health

75

standpoint? The most dangerous steroids, according to one expert, are the type that Brian Bosworth had in his bloodstream—a nandroline preparation called Deca-Durabolin, charged Dr. Donald H. Catlin, an NCAA drug-testing expert and director of UCLA's Paul Ziffren Olympic Analytical Laboratory. "Nandroline is the most dangerous of the steroids," said Catlin. "It's administered in an oil-based solution and releases its contents over weeks and months; consequently the pituitary is suppressed for a long time. My clinical impression is that if one had to take steroids, the oral agents are less medically dangerous than the oil-based injected solutions."[10]

'Roid Rage

Many athletes claim that they feel more aggressive when on a cycle of steroids. A study at McLean Hospital in Belmont, Massachusetts, found that five of forty-one individuals reported "psychotic symptoms" while using steroids, as opposed to none when not on them. Others reported "a manic episode during steroid use . . . and major depression."[11]

"It changes you; it makes you an ego monster," former University of South Carolina football player Tommy Chaikin told the *Los Angeles Times*.[12] For a while Chaikin said he felt "godlike" and "invincible."

His reaction is fairly typical. Many athletes who use steroids, including the majority of women in one published study, say they believe the aggressive self they become on drugs is an asset during competition, although it may damage family life and normal interaction with people.[13]

Users may fly off the handle without provocation. Young men have been known to start fistfights without reason, punch lockers and walls, jump up and down on car trunks, and seriously injure other people while in the midst of a 'roid rage. "Any little thing could set you off," a New York dealer told reporter Mark Kriegel when he sold him Anadrol-50.[14]

Unfortunately, there is no way to predict whom steroids will set off. Normally subdued and quiet people may get only slightly more aggressive on steroids. Then again, they might try to take off the head of someone who bumps into them on the street.

Onetime steroid user Ken Matlob had to leave his home as a teenager because he started so many quarrels with family members. He once destroyed another man's car with his bare hands and a knife. He frequently injured himself, punching brick walls and banging his head into a metal cabinet. Another time he broke a man's nose.[15]

Steroid users often report that their judgment becomes warped and that they do things their social conscience otherwise wouldn't let them do. One youth recalled a night when he got drunk after injecting steroids and went out with a friend who had a pistol. Not content with blasting street signs, they went out into the country and shot a cow. Another time he knocked down a delivery boy and held a loaded shotgun to his head.[16] Would steroid users act the same way without the drugs? More research is definitely needed in this area.

Steroid-related killings and assaults have been common enough that attorneys have defended their clients with the argument that they were not fully aware of what they were doing when they committed a crime in the midst of a steroid rage. For example, in a Florida trial, a twenty-three-year-old bodybuilder pleaded that "steroid psychosis" caused him to beat a hitchhiker to death.

How Do Steroids Affect Females?

While aggressiveness and hypertension (due to sodium and fluid retention) are common complaints of both male and female steroid users, there are some characteristics and hazards peculiar to each sex.

Girls and women notice that their voices become deeper and more masculine. They may suffer balding and irregular menstrual cycles or see an increase in facial and body hair. Women often report enlargement of the clitoris, noted Dr. Michael A. Nelson.

Dr. Richard H. Strauss interviewed women steroid users who reported breast shrinkage, decreased body fat, increased appetite, cessation of menstruation, increased libido, and general masculinization of their bodies.

One of the unknowns in steroid use by women is whether or not the drug can adversely affect the health of their future children. "I wonder if I'll have a normal child," said onetime steroid user Diane Williams, a sprinter on the 1984 Olympic team who has admitted that her body acquired "male characteristics" from long-term use of the drug from 1981 to 1984.[17] Additional studies over time should answer whether steroids affect a woman's ability to conceive and whether or not, over an extended period of time, undesirable male characteristics in women may diminish or disappear when steroid use is halted.

How Steroids
Affect Males

Men report a shrinking of the testicles after using steroids. Ironically, by injecting or orally taking testosterone for a prolonged time period, a male athlete's own testosterone and sperm-count levels drop to very low levels. Ben Johnson's tests during the 1988 Olympics showed his natural testosterone level had plunged dramatically.

Both impotence and temporary sterility have been reported by male steroid users. Whether long-term sterility will dog these men remains to be seen. Permanent baldness has been reported by many steroid users, but it is impossible to say with certainty how many might have lost their hair anyway.

In addition, according to Dr. Gabe Mirkin, the worst-case scenarios for males who abuse steroids are heart attacks, sterility, tumors, and liver cancer.[18] Whether such problems would have arisen anyway is a matter of speculation.

Health Problems
Common to Both Sexes

What is known about extended use of oral steroids is that they can interfere with liver function and lead to biliary obstruction, jaundice, and slow-growing liver tumors—all of which are reversible if steroid use is halted, reported the *American Journal of Nursing.* "Though rare, blood-filled sacs [peliosis hepatitis] can form in the liver and rupture, causing hemorrhage, liver failure and death."

The journal advised steroid-using athletes to seek medical help at once if any of the following symptoms of liver damage are noted: jaundice, white or clay-colored bowel movements, and deep-orange-colored urine.[19]

What Are the Signs
of a Steroid User?

Unfortunately, many columnists believe themselves experts on steroids. "Steroid use may have become a cancer in our sports, but it's no mystery in terms of detection," wrote *Houston Chronicle* columnist Ed Fowler. "In most cases, the signs are external and readily apparent—from inordinate muscle growth to acne on the back and shoulders."

Inordinate size and strength are *not* clear indications of steroid use—although a massive gain over a brief time span is a telltale sign—because some genetically gifted athletes have both. In addition, many teenage athletes who take no drugs whatsoever have acne problems.

Many gifted athletes today are unfairly accused of cheating simply because of impressive builds they've cultivated with proper nutrition, hard work, and superior training techniques.

79

Many players, however, show no short-term exterior differences other than more refined body definition. High school coaches, in particular, say they have difficulty spotting steroid users because adolescents often grow taller and bulkier in spurts. Notre Dame strength coach Scott Raridon, a former football teammate at the University of Nebraska of admitted steroid user Dean Steinkuhler, saw no signs that Steinkuhler used steroids. "I played right next to the guy and never knew," said Raridon.[20]

But the acne and the rapid gains in bulk may be significant. In addition, other telltale signs of steroid use include yellow eyes from the drug's toxic effect on the liver, shiny skin, difficulty in urinating, elevated blood pressure and too rapid a heartbeat, breasts in men, premature balding, facial bumps and acne, mood shifts, and, in women, masculine voices, male-shaped torsos, and sudden growth of body hair.

Some steroid users, however, do not suffer apparent adverse effects other than an aroused (or sometimes repressed) libido and a tendency toward being more aggressive than usual. At present, it is impossible to predict which steroid users will later develop health problems, although it's clear that athletes who take massive overdoses, such as football player Steve Courson, are playing Russian roulette with their own lives.

Another problem with taking steroids is that while certain negative side effects such as mood swings stop when a user quits, like cigarettes, the steroids are often difficult to give up. Whether or not steroids are physically addicting (and one recent study indicates they may be, see page 82) they do tend to create a psychological addiction. People who perform better or develop bigger builds on steroids are unwilling to lose the edge once they have it. Yet that is precisely what happens when a steroid user quits cold.

"Bulging biceps and ham-hock thighs do a fast fade

when the chemicals are halted," said writer Anastasia Toufexis in *Time.* "So do the feelings of being powerful and manly. Almost every user winds up back on the drugs. A self-image that relies on a steroid-soaked body may be difficult to change."

There is one terribly unfunny irony about steroids. If a former steroid user requires a new heart or kidney, the drug of choice to keep the host body from rejecting the new organ is cortical adrenal steroids. If Steve Courson is able to find a heart donor, he will need drugs related to steroids to recover.

"I've gone from dominant football player to cardio invalid," he admitted to *USA Today.* "I just don't know if the same chemicals helped me become both."

Additional Problems with
Black-Market Drugs

Even physicians who felt that steroid use posed only minimal risks if athletes followed their instructions expressed severe reservations about black-market steroids.

The quality of black-market steroids is uncertain at best. There is no guarantee that steroids are correctly labeled, that they haven't been adulterated, and that the recommended dosages are accurate.

Illegal supplies come from clandestine, unlicensed laboratories all over the world, including the United States, Mexico, Europe, and South America. There is no one to regulate the purity of materials or to insist that the drugs be manufactured in a sterile environment. Many athletes actually finance training periods overseas by bringing steroids back with them to resell stateside.

Contrary to locker-room folklore, the chances that the consumer will get steroid products inferior to those sold by legitimate drug companies are quite high. The *New York Times* estimates that 95 percent of all black-market steroids are counterfeit.[21]

Without a doubt, a steroid user is safer getting steroids from a physician, but in doing so, the athlete must ask the doctor to break the law. One of the problems associated with steroids' becoming a controlled substance is that as the drugs become harder to get and the demand rises, black-market peddlers will grow wealthier.

Can Steroids
Be Addicting?

In December 1989, the results of a study were published that suggested that steroid users may become addicted to the drugs. The study was contested by other researchers who believe steroids may cause strong psychological dependence but are not addicting.

Kenneth B. Kashkin, Ph.D, of Yale University School of Medicine, said that when people try to break the steroid habit, "there can be symptoms of acute withdrawal, similar to withdrawal from alcohol—anxiety, irritability, insomnia, hot and cold flashes, and muscle aches." He also observed delayed depression, including thoughts of suicide, like that seen after cocaine withdrawal.[22]

In conclusion, Professor Kashkin and fellow researcher Herbert D. Kleber, Ph.D., said that while steroids cannot be classified as pleasure drugs, their use results in similar disturbances: use over longer periods than desired, unsuccessful attempts to stop, substantial time spent obtaining, using, or recovering from the substance, and withdrawal symptoms upon stopping.[23]

6
DRUG TESTING

Why Test?

The theories behind requiring drug tests for athletes are simple:

1. The abuses of street and performance-enhancing drugs have reached such a magnitude that users need to be protected from themselves.

2. Because nonusers in athletics are put at a competitive disadvantage—and may even be said to be in danger of being hurt by aggressive steroid users in such sports as football—something has to be done to help the innocent athletes who compete chemical-free.

3. People may be less tempted to start or continue drug use if they know they are to be tested and disqualified for using steroids or street drugs. Many experts feel the only effec-

tive deterrent for steroid abuse is banishment from sport. Hurdler Edwin Moses and other athletes have gone on record as saying that abuse will continue as long as the powers that be punish only athletes such as Ben Johnson for their indiscretion. Johnson's shame and embarrassment as he fell from glory overnight were painful for the public to watch on television—all the more so since his advisers escaped the ridicule he had to face alone. Moses recommends that "all doctors, coaches, trainers and managers who assist an athlete in taking drugs be subject to punishment" as well as athletes, "the last link in the chain."[1]

Indeed, many athletes have expressed indignation over the way Ben Johnson's reputation was shattered after he tested positive for steroids. "The punishments and the crimes don't seem to fit," complained 1976 gold medalist (discus) Mac Wilkins. "Ben Johnson took drugs to improve his athletic performance, and he's gone through hell. . . . You'd think he blew up a whole town and killed a million people, the way everyone's reacting."[2]

Drug testing in the workplace, in all NCAA college sports, and in many professional sports is done often enough now to be called commonplace. The trend of the 1990s, however, will be drug testing of athletes for street and performance-enhancing drugs in the high schools as well.

Drug testing of high school athletes is now a reality. Two institutions in Tippecanoe County, Indiana, have received permission of a federal court that ruled it is constitutional to test cheerleaders and athletes for drug use. Testing began on a regular basis in August 1989, and students caught the first time were to be suspended

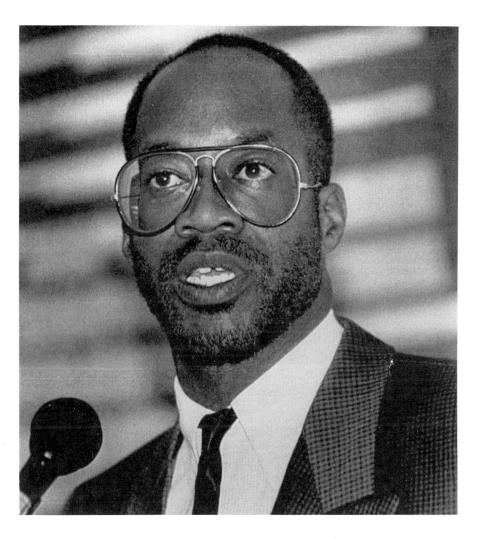

*Edwin Moses, U.S. two-time gold medalist
hurdler, speaking before a gathering at the
National Steroid Consensus Meeting in 1989.
He felt that a drug-testing program in track
and field was "much needed" and that steroid
use must be "cleaned up" by educating
athletes on the dangers of steroid use.*

for several games and given professional counseling. Harsher penalties were to be given repeat offenders.

And in 1989 the NFL finally announced twenty-three one-month suspensions for players who tested positive for steroids, although some observers said that the announced testing allowed too many offenders to escape undetected. Tests were conducted in training camps, allowing time for most users to clear their systems of banned substances. "We're not anxious to catch anyone," said the then NFL commissioner Pete Rozelle. "We simply want them to stop using steroids."

The Case Against
Drug Testing
Those opposed to the testing of steroids offer six main arguments:

They argue that insufficient medical research is available to categorically ban steroid users.

They argue that if you legislate against steroids you need to legislate against tobacco and alcohol and other health-threatening substances.

They argue that college athletes, top amateurs, and professionals who are eighteen should be able to make their own decisions on steroid use.

They believe that it is unfair to single out athletes and cheerleaders for drug-abuse tests. "Mandatory urinalysis is an invasion of privacy," insists Norma Rollins of the New York Civil Liberties Union.[3] Those opposed argue that at the high school and college level nonathletes should also be tested. A major sore-point is that coaches—including beefy strength coaches—are not tested along with their athletes.

They say that the privacy of the innocent and rights of the innocent will be trod upon to find the guilty. "I thought we had certain rights," complained pro-football player Jerry Bell. "I don't feel like I have to prove I'm not on drugs."[4]

They argue that the very act of banning a substance creates a black market for those who think the risk of getting caught is worth the profits they make.

"There would be no black market in steroids if there were no bans against their possession and use," argued *USA Today* guest columnist Jeff Riggenbach. "This is the invariable outcome of attempts to protect people from themselves by interfering in their business, denying them freedom to make their own decisions and placing prohibitions on substances or activities they have decided to make a part of their lives."[5]

Kate Schmidt, a onetime world-record holder in the women's javelin event who has said she never used steroids, believes it is foolish to test athletes for drug use to protect their health. She noted that anyone who competes in sports at a top level usually comes away with severe chronic injuries, even without taking drugs.

"In my case, a rewarding, exciting athletic career has left me with the right shoulder of a sixty-five-year-old woman," a then thirty-two-year-old Schmidt told *Sports Illustrated*. "For many years I practiced and competed through considerable pain. No TAC [The Athletics Congress] official, though, tried to keep me out of the Olympics "for my own good."

Schmidt's suggestion is to reduce the pressures in sports to win at any cost that cause athletes to use drugs in the first place. "Then perhaps we can return to the true joys of sport," she concluded.

Those who oppose testing frequently say that education is the solution, but drug expert Sam McDowell, a recovering alcoholic and former big league pitcher, cautions that there are no shortcut answers. "So many educators get all hot for drug education, and they'll bring in some hot-shot athlete or movie star, and he may talk a couple of hours on drug abuse and tell his own experience, and that's it," McDowell complained to the *Dallas Morning News*.

McDowell then called for a long-term approach to drug education, suggesting that students take required classes in the subject. "If a student flunks the course, he would have to take it over again in summer school, just like biology or physics," he said. "Some people might say we're panicking. But if we began right now, working to get the program mandatory in all states and added to every school curriculum, we're still talking twenty-five years before it's all functioning properly."[6]

The Case
for Testing

The major obstacle to drug testing long had been that monitored urine or blood-collecting tests violated an athlete's right to privacy. But nearly all judicial rulings in recent years have been similar to that of a U.S. District Court judge who in February 1988 "ruled that the privacy issue is outweighed by the need to protect student-athletes' health, reduce temptation to use drugs, and ensure fair competitions."[7]

Few college coaches have taken stands against the ruling—even those who in the past knew or suspected they had steroid users on their teams.

Every football coach in the Big Ten, for example, has recommended that the conference administer tests to detect anabolic steroid use. According to the *NCAA*

News, the ten coaches reasoned that such testing is necessary to "eliminate innuendo about who is taking what, clear the reputation of players who have been wrongly accused of taking steroids, and ensure that teams are competing on the same level."[8]

A similar rationale for depriving athletes of what would be considered a civil right was given to United Press International by University of Connecticut athletic director Todd Turner when he announced the university's decision to endorse drug testing. "I certainly don't like the idea of drug testing, and I personally find it disappointing that we have to resort to this, but our athletes want to be free of the suspicion of drug abuse."[9]

For several years, while drug testing was in its infancy, charges and countercharges flourished that many steroid-using athletes simply were getting friends and "clean" teammates to take the tests for them. Without doubt, there were some abuses. One expert has said that improper administering of tests results in urine samples that are worthless.

"If samples were not collected properly, they might as well not be analyzed," said Dr. Donald H. Catlin, an NCAA drug tester and chief of the Division of Clinical Pharmacology at UCLA. "There is no way I could justify working on samples that could have come from anywhere."[10]

The Case for
Random Testing

Even the onetime prescriber of anabolic steroids to athletes, Dr. Robert Kerr, recommends frequent testing as the only means of combating cheating with drugs. However, he said that testing athletes in competition is not the best way of locating guilty parties. "Some of these drugs can be out of the system in days," said Dr. Kerr. "You've got to have a way to [test] the athletes when they're out training."[11]

Miler Steve Scott charged that much of the drug testing done by colleges is a costly joke, anyway, because they lie and cover up to protect their athletes and the image of their institutions. "Have the NCAA do it," argued Scott. "Don't leave it up to the schools, because they won't bust their own people."[12]

Other experts and athletes say that those who test for drugs must increase their knowledge to be able to ferret out increasingly sophisticated steroid users. "I was at the Fiesta Bowl, and I'm seeing the players walk down the hallways and they're behemoths," grumbled Steve Scott, one of the foremost milers in history. "They do their little drug test at a bowl game and everyone's clean. Well, of course, they're going to be clean; they know what they're doing [in disguising steroid use]. They have it [down] to a science. If they really want to address the drug problem, they should have random drug testing at every game in college."[13]

During the 1986 postseason bowl testing, twenty-one NCAA football players tested positive for drug use and were ruled ineligible. The biggest story was the suspension of University of Oklahoma star Brian Bosworth. In contrast, at the conclusion of the 1988 season not one violation was detected; but many experts felt it was only because steroid users had plenty of opportunity to mask the substance. One of the most successful masking agents was a drug called probenecid. It is now one of more than 100 banned substances tested for by the IOC.

Bill Mallory, head football coach at Indiana University, agreed. He recommended that testing "be done through the whole year unannounced, or these guys could drain it out of their system."[14]

One athlete likened today's drug testing at major competitions to a speed trap "that everyone in town knows about." The athletes go full speed until they reach the danger zone where they're just about to be caught and then drive slowly and safely and smugly past the enforcement agencies.[15]

Some steroids pass very quickly through the system. Duncan Atwood, a javelin thrower suspended for eighteen months for steroid use in 1986, said there are drugs "that wash out in three days."[16]

Clearly, at the college and high school level, the answer to detecting users is when they are unprepared, in random testing in the off-season, and at all times during a season, not only prior to bowl games. At present, many amateur track competitors simply fail to show up at a competition if word filters through to them that there will be testing.

Without much doubt, the NCAA will ask its members to consider adopting random testing on other than the present voluntary basis. Whether certain schools known for having steroid problems, such as the University of South Carolina, will vote to approve such a measure remains to be seen.

What is likely to be approved, however, are team sanctions against universities that have individuals who flunk their drug tests. At the present writing, the issue is under discussion.

What Is Tested?

Amateur and professional players are tested for known substances that most international drug-testing laboratories are familiar with. However, many experts charge that sophisticated coaches and athletes know of performance-aiding substances that tests cannot detect. Visit any major gym in a large city and you'll hear shop-talk about the latest performance-enhancing drug that isn't yet on the banned list.

In fact, the athletic world was just as shocked by Ben Johnson's positive test for anabolic steroids as was the general public—but for a far different reason. What amazed Johnson's fellow athletes was how he could be so stupid or careless to allow himself to get nabbed. "In 1988, being a drug-enhanced athlete is disgustingly simple," renowned Olympic hurdler Edwin Moses told *Newsweek.*[17]

Most experts believe that more than 50 percent of Olympic athletes have had some experience with banned drugs. They insist that it is naive to think that the 6 percent of NFL players who tested positive in 1988 for steroid use are the only men in the league "juicing up," as users call it.

Testing procedures are fairly consistent for all sporting events. Following a football game, an NCAA Final Four game, or an Olympic race, athletes leave the cheering crowds for the unglamorous and somewhat embarrassing purpose of entering a designated rest room to urinate into a specimen bottle. A portion of the specimen is taken to a chemist for immediate testing, and a portion is refrigerated for later examination if that first test should be labeled positive.

One of the best explanations of how drug testing catches cheaters was given by *U.S. News & World Report.* "The big gun in any lab's arsenal is a two-step procedure called gas chromatography/mass spectrometry. In the first stage, a sample of urine is injected into a special, heated column that separates the liquid into its chemical constituents. Each substance takes a characteristic amount of time to pass through the column. Small molecules such as water travel more quickly than bulky steroids. In the second stage, the emerging chemicals are bombarded by electrons. Unlike dinner plates, molecules shatter into predictable pieces. A computer program analyzes the molecular debris and, with the aid of a vast, stored atlas of substances, makes positive identification."[18]

When athletes test positive, they are requested to witness a retesting that is done on the remainder of the original specimen. Some scientists say that testing is foolproof and sufficient evidence to label an athlete as a cheater. Other scientists and experts disagree. Swedish doctor Arne Ljungqvist, a member of the IOC Medical Commission, admitted that it is sometimes difficult to interpret test results, even for professionals. "The result of an analysis is not like a sheet of paper which says positive or negative, but an analytical data which requires a specialist['s] evaluation. In most cases, it's quite clear that a sample contains a banned substance and in other cases it's not."[19]

And as Dr. Park Jong Sei, director of Olympic drug testing in Seoul at the 1988 Olympics, admitted to *The New York Times*, "In one or two cases. . . . I thought the athlete had used drugs for performance enhancement [but] the majority overruled me."[20]

Is Testing
Foolproof?

The strongest argument against drug testing is that no system is 100 percent foolproof. Administrators at all levels of sports cringe at the thought of an innocent athlete being judged a drug user. More likely, however, they regret knowing that so many guilty parties have beaten the system, using *legal* prescription drugs, for example, to "mask" the presence of steroids in their bodies.

Mistakes have been made. In April 1989, for example, the IOC suspended seven prominent drug-testing laboratories from its approved list because they were judged at least partially unreliable for committing "some small mistakes," including administrative errors, a failure to detect steroid users, and insufficient written analysis of tests conducted. The laboratories—located in such far-flung nations as the United States, Canada, the Soviet Union, and Finland—were given slap-on-the-wrist penalties of four months' suspension. "In some

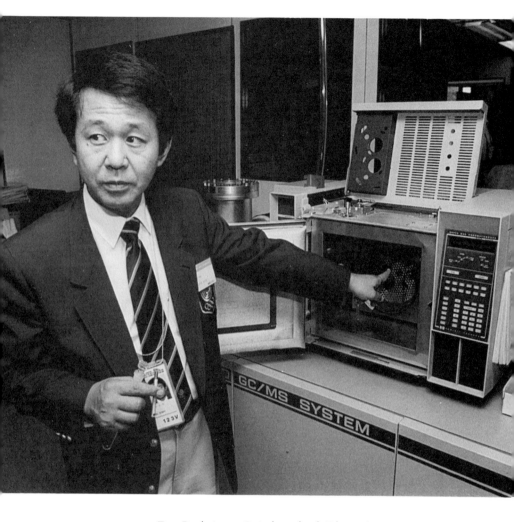

Dr. Park Jong-Sei, head of Olympic drug testing in 1988, points at a gas chromatograph, a drug-test system connected to a computer terminal that will analyze and display the results on a screen. All Olympic competitors must go through this test.

cases only one small mistake was made, but we cannot allow even one," said Prince Alexander de Merode, chairperson of the IOC's medical commission. "IOC labs must be perfect in drug detection."[21]

But one day a test that is 100 percent effective may be found. The best new procedure to detect "blood doping" is to analyze blood samples. Blood doping—the practice of removing a pint of blood from an athlete, pumping it full of oxygen, and replacing it just before an event—heretofore was undetectable in the usual urine tests. Consequently, athletes cheating in events such as cross-country skiing and bicycling were never caught by standard tests.

During the 1990s, a combination of urine and blood testing may become the norm at such important competitions as the Olympics. According to Dr. James Stray-Gunderson, U.S. Ski Team physician, testing both urine and blood "can really nail down the picture of what this [athlete] has been doing with hormones."[22] Also in the testing stage is a test for drug use by microscopic examination of human hair, a method that is less demeaning than urine testing and less objectionable than blood testing.

There is no question that the major change in the drug picture in the last decade of the century is that steroid research will at last catch up to the reality of its use in both amateur and professional sports. Along the way, there will be smeared reputations, bitter recriminations, and demands that the records of convicted steroid users be erased. Steroids have been the biggest controversy in sports during the 1980s, and there is little reason to think that it will cease to be a hot issue as mandatory, random drug-testing legislation is enacted at all levels of sport and, perhaps, society.

One of the biggest problems that athletic programs on the high school and college level must face is that a well-executed drug program can cost as much as $100–$200 per player.

"It's going to be expensive," said former Michigan coach Bo Schembechler, "but we've got to stamp this thing out."[23]

His former nemesis, Michigan State University football coach George Perles, agreed, saying that getting rid of steroids was his number-one priority, "even if we lose every game."[24]

AFTERWORD

Life After
Steroid Testing

Advocates of steroids and those who condemn them have little common ground on which to meet. The medical and scientific communities have tried their best for years to discourage athletes, fitness buffs, and the general public from taking steroids. On the other hand, those athletes who have taken steroids, with few or no short-term side effects, swear that steroids work and that the athlete should not be punished.

But the spread of drug testing by 1989 through high school, college, amateur, and professional sports has left little doubt that the day when a steroid user could "juice up" with impunity is long gone. In fact, as more and more powers that be adopt random testing, the percentage of steroid users will continue to drop, although there will still be some who feel the opportunities to enhance performance through chemicals are worth the health consequences and the risks associated with getting caught and branded a steroid user.

Without question, athletes who use steroids stand an undetermined statistical chance of suffering negative physical effects. A healthy male bodybuilder developed liver cancer after using steroids, says the American College of Sports Medicine. An East Berlin defector named Renate Neufeld complained that steroid use had ruined her sprinting career, making her barely able to walk. Swedish discus medalist Donald McCormick charged in 1978 that steroids had eroded his calcium and caused him to require six knee operations.[1] Other athletes have grown muscles too big for their tendons, resulting in painful and debilitating tearing.

While it is pointless to speculate on just what percentage of athletes will continue to take steroids, there seems to be no question that the substances will continue to sell on the black market to adolescents and others who desire the size and strength that steroids can provide.

With so many drawbacks to consider, the best alternative remains the "natural" way to train. The honest approach will always appeal to athletes who want to keep their health and integrity—both today and in the future—as well as good builds. For such athletes, there are any number of sources to consult in terms of workout and nutritional programs.

Many experts claim that natural methods to build strength and size are still the most desirable. It will be interesting to note whether there will be a reduction in the number of "wide bodies" in the NFL and the Olympics as a result of heightened awareness of the dangers of steroid use and the prevalence of drug testing.

The Olympic 100-meter and long-jump champion Carl Lewis said that he thought it was a "blessing" that Ben Johnson and other athletes have been caught using steroids. "We have to advance the sport, and advancing the sport only comes by fighting things detrimental to it," he said.[2]

"It just doesn't smack of good health to me: liver disease, impotency, other diseases," agreed Chicago Bear strength coordinator Clyde Emrich. "In football, it seems to me that strength does not become a substitute for skills anyway. I'm just happy that the league has the backbone to enforce its policy against steroid use."[3]

If you're serious about improving your size, strength, and athletic performance without chemicals, you'd be wise to see what is available in your area of the country in terms of a program specializing in free weights. Such a program takes time, unlike combining free weights with steroid use, but the effects are rewarding. You'll be happier and your build won't disappear when you've gotten off steroids.

To begin, men and women should visit a doctor to make certain that their bodies are healthy enough to sustain the rigors of a full-scale fitness program.

You'll want to keep a record of your aerobic performances. Those men and women who opt to try weight lifting should also record their improvement from week to week. There is a feeling of satisfaction in hoisting more and more iron and knowing that physical gains have been made without cheating.

Lifters should be certain to give their bodies a good overall workout. There's no sense in having a fine caboose if a locomotive can't budge it.

Find a program that allows you to exercise your arms, both biceps and triceps, chest ("pecs" in lifters' terms), back, and legs ("quadriceps"). You'll get the most benefit from performing eight to twelve repetitions in all areas of the body you exercise as well as by giving your body time to recuperate from workouts, advised Tom Deters, managing publisher of *Muscle and Fitness.*

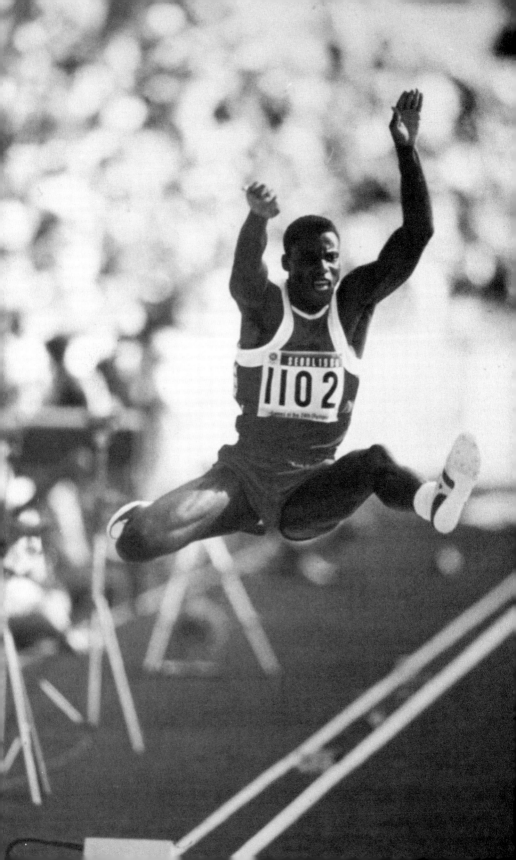

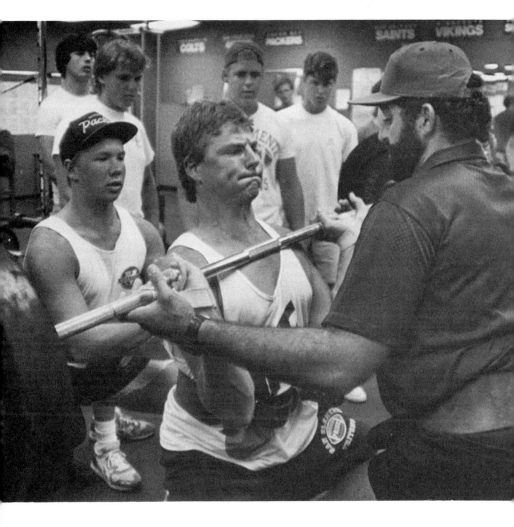

*Left: Carl Lewis, U.S. Olympic gold medal
winner in both the 100-meter and long-jump
track and field competitions in 1988.*

*Above: grunting with effort, a high school
football player attempts to qualify in
weight lifting in San Clemente, California.*

"Every rep[etition] has to be 100 percent effort," said Deters. "Otherwise you're just going through the motions. No bouncing, no cheating."[4]

Nutritional Solutions

Also, good nutrition is a must. You'll need to break the "fast food" habit and give up sodas and snack food—particularly late at night, when they do the most harm. If you eat properly, you won't need protein powders and diet supplements, which have been attacked enough in print to merit another book such as this one. It goes without saying that cigarettes, alcohol, and drugs have no place in the life of someone trying to build the best possible body.

"The key is nutrition," said University of Nebraska strength coach Boyd Epley, who claims to have no respect for "goof-ball power lifters" who use steroids. "If you're selective in the food that you eat, you can make the same gains [weight and strength] naturally as long as your workouts are intense. . . . My job at Nebraska isn't to build strength that will be displayed in a one-lift rep, it's to help these athletes attain the best possible balance of strength and speed."[5]

The old maxim of eating breakfast like a king, lunch like a prince, and supper like a pauper is a wise one to follow because it makes most efficient use of the body's metabolism. Workout expert Tom Deters's recommendation is that a bodybuilder's diet should consist of 15 percent fat, 25 percent protein, and 60 percent carbohydrates. He also recommends that you should give your body "solid, uninterrupted sleep" at roughly the same time every night and keep your existence as stress-free as possible.[6]

In the future, because scientists, coaches, and athletes from all nations are looking for healthy alternatives to steroids to help build size, strength, and performance, there may be substitutes for anabolic steroids—although there may never be a drug that gives such quick results to certain athletes. However, as long as a quick buck is to be made, there will be those who offer "instant" and "easy" ways to build better bodies. Guard against such hucksters.

If you are currently using steroids and you wish to get involved in alternate programs to help you get off steroids yet keep some of the gains your body has made with chemicals, there are organizations offering help.

The Chicago College of Osteopathic Medicine has set up a steroid help center for anyone with questions, said Dr. Bob Goldman, author of *Death in the Locker Room.* The telephone number is (312) 515-6100. Another valuable source is local doctors who practice sports medicine, although they, of course, charge for consultations.

Lists of safe medications and banned drugs are available from the International Olympic Committee (IOC), Chateau de Vidy 1007, Lausanne, Switzerland.

A hot line open 8:00 A.M. to 5:00 P.M. (Mountain Time zone) is available for questions on steroids, medication, and banned substances. The source is the U.S. Olympic Committee (USOC), and its toll-free phone number is (1-800) 233-0393. The committee advises athletes, coaches, trainers, and the physicians who work with these athletes.

To report a steroid seller, contact your local law enforcement agency or the Department of Justice, Drug Enforcement Administration, 400 Sixth Street S.W., Washington, D.C. 20024.

Consult your librarian for the address of state athletic commissions that often have pamphlets on the subject. New York State's Athletic Commission, for example, is located at 270 Broadway, New York, NY 10007.

To obtain information and pamphlets (small charge) on steroids and other subjects, write the American College of Sports Medicine, P.O. Box 1440, Indianapolis, IN 46206-1440. The telephone number is (317) 637-9200.

For booklets and a list of banned substances called "Doping Control Regulations," contact the International Amateur Athletic Federation (IAFF), 3 Hans Crescent, London SW1. The telephone number in London is (01) 581-8771.

For pamphlets (inquire if there is a charge for publications or handling) frankly discussing steroids and other banned substances, contact the following organizations:

United States Department of Education
Attention: The Challenge Program
Seventh and D Streets
Washington, DC 20202

National Basketball Association
Attention: Don't Foul Out program
645 Fifth Ave.
New York, NY 10022

Drug Abuse Council, Inc.
1828 L Street N.W.
Washington, DC 20036

The Athletics Congress (TAC)
5 West Sixty-third Street
New York, NY 10023

National Institute on Drug Abuse
5600 Fishers Lane
Rockville, MD 20857

Public Affairs Pamphlets
381 Park Avenue South
New York, NY 10016

National Council on Drug Abuse
571 West Jackson Avenue
Chicago, IL 60606

National Hockey League
Attention: Public Relations Department
650 Fifth Avenue, Floor 33
New York, NY 10019

National Clearinghouse for
Drug Abuse Information
P.O. Box 416
Kensington, MD 20795

SOURCE NOTES

Chapter One

1. *USA Today,* 15 June 1989, 9C.

2. Natalie Angier, "The Case Against Steroids," *Discover,* November 1983, p. 98.

3. The *New York Times,* 17 November 1988, p. D31.

4. Michael A. Nelson, "Androgenic-Anabolic Steroid Use in Adolescents," *Journal of Pediatric Health Care* 3 July-August (1989): 175; Gabe Mirkin "Hormonal Helpers," *Health,* March 1984, p. 6.

5. Ibid.

6. Tim Walker, "Bulk Power," *Expo,* Spring 1986, p. 11.

7. Syndicated column by Charles E. Yesalis, the *New York Times* syndicate, "Steroids Enhance Muscularity and Physical Capabilities," as it appeared in the *Ann Arbor News,* 27 February 1989, p. F12.

8. *Newsweek,* 10 October 1988, p. 56.

9. Nelson, *Journal of Pediatric Health Care,* pp. 176, 179.

10. *Hammond Times,* 12 March 1989, p. A-18.

11. Walker, *Expo,* p. 11.

12. Richard H. Straus, Mariah T. Liggett, and Richard R. Lanese, "Anabolic Steroid Use and Perceived Effects in Ten Weight-Trained Women Athletes," *Journal of the American Medical Association* 253 (1985): 2871.

13. William Oscar Johnson, "Steroids: A Problem of Huge Dimensions," *Sports Illustrated,* 13 May 1985, p. 54.

14. The *New York Times,* 18 November 1988, p. A22.

15. Quoted in *NCAA News,* 12 April 1989, p. 5.

16. Syndicated column by Mike Barnes for United Press International, as it appeared in *NCAA News,* 18 January 1989, p. 4.

17. *NCAA News,* 19 July 1989, p. 4.

18. Eric Mishara, "Dead Russian Athletes," *Omni,* 8 March 1986, p. 30.

19. Information summarized from Bob Goldman's *Death in the Locker Room,* chap. 1 (South Bend: Icarus Press, 1984).

20. *USA Today,* 11 April 1989, p. 10A.

21. *Newsweek,* 10 October 1988, p. 57.

22. *NCAA News,* 12 April 1989, p. 8

23. *USA Today,* 11 April 1989, p. 10A.

Chapter Two

1. Nelson, *Journal of Pediatric Health Care,* p. 176.

2. Strauss, et al., *JAMA,* p. 2872.

3. Johnson, *Sports Illustrated,* p. 52.

4. Nelson, p. 176.

5. Strauss, p. 2871.

6. *USA Today,* 20 June 1989, p. 10C.

7. Ibid.

8. *U.S. News & World Report,* 10 October 1988, p. 39.

9. Unsigned article, "Of Steroids and Sports," *Emergency Medicine,* 15 February 1988, p. 206.

10. The *New York Times,* 18 November 1922, p. A22.

11. *Muncie Star,* 12 March 1989, p. 15A.

12. *NCAA News,* 26 April 1989, p. 4.

13. Ibid.

14. The *New York Times,* 18 November 1988, p. 1A.

15. Walker, *Expo,* p. 11.

16. Johnson, *Sports Illustrated,* p. 50.

17. Armen Keteyian, "A Business Built on Bulk," *Sports Illustrated,* 13 May 1985, p. 61.

Chapter Three
1. The *New York Times,* 20 November 1988, p. 34.

2. *NCAA News,* 19 July 1989, p. 4.

3. *USA Today,* 5 July 1989, p. 2C.

4. The Gannett News Service as reprinted in *NCAA News,* 2 August 1989, p. 2.

5. *NCAA News, 2 August 1989, p. 20.*

6. *USA Today,* 9 March 1989, p. 3C.

7. *NCAA News, 2 August 1989, p. 4.*

8. Michael A. Nelson, "Androgenic-Anabolic Steroid Use in Adolescents," *Journal of Pediatric Health Care* 3 July (1989): 175.

9. Herbert A. Haupt and George D. Rovere, "Anabolic Steroids: A Review of the Literature," *American Journal of Sports Medicine* 12 (1984): 475

10. *USA Today,* 12 July 1989, p. 1C.

11. *Hammond Times,* 14 March 1989, p. A-12.

12. *USA Today,* 20 June 1989, Section C, p. 1.
13. *USA Today,* 6 April 1989, p. 10C.
14. Ibid.
15. *NCAA News,* 10 May 1989, p. 4.
16. Ibid.
17. *USA Today,* 20 June 1989, 1C.
18. William Oscar Johnson, "Hit for a Loss," *Sports Illustrated,* 19 September 1988, p. 52.
19. *Washington Post,* 10 May 1989, p. 1.
20. Syndicated column by Mike Barnes, United Press International, as it appeared in *NCAA News,* 18 January 1989, p. 4.

Chapter Four
1. Syndicated the *New York Times* column carried by *Ann Arbor News,* 27 February 1989, p. F12.
2. *Chicago Sun-Times,* "Steroids: A Special Section," February 1989.
3. Ibid.
4. *Time,* 30 January 1989, p. 78.
5. Ibid.
6. *Chicago Sun-Times,* "Steroids: A Special Section," February 1989.
7. Ibid.
8. *Chicago Sun-Times,* February 1989, p. 1.
9. Ibid.
10. *USA Today,* 13 July 1989, p. 1C.
11. *USA Today,* 24 March 1989, p. 2C.
12. 1989 Patricia McLaughlin/United Press Syndicate.
13. *USA Today,* 6 April 1989, p. 10C.

14. Syndicated column distributed by The *New York Times* syndicate, as it appeared in *Ann Arbor News,* 27 February 1989, p. F12.

15. *Post-Tribune,* 16 December 1988, p. A-3.

16. *Men's Fitness,* August 1988, p. 123.

17. The *New York Times,* 18 November 1988, p. 1A.

18. *Chicago Sun-Times,* "Steroids: A Special Section," February 1989.

Chapter Five

1. *USA Today,* 5 July 1989, p. 1C.

2. Associated Press wire, 10 July 1989.

3. The *New York Times,* 20 November 1988, p. 34.

4. *Time,* 30 January 1989, p. 78.

5. *Newsweek,* 10 October 1988, p. 57.

6. *USA Today,* 11 April 1989, p. 10A.

7. *USA Today,* 5 July 1989, p. 2C.

8. *Sports Illustrated,* 10 November 1986, p. 18.

9. *USA Today,* 23 January 1987, p. 6C.

10. *Journal of the American Medical Association,* 23 and 30 January 1987, p. 421.

11. The *New York Times,* 20 November 1988, p. 34.

12. *NCAA News,* 12 April 1989, p. 5.

13. Ibid.

14. *Daily News,* 25 June 1989, p. 28.

15. *Chicago Sun-Times,* February 1989, p. 5.

16. Tommy Chaikin with Rick Telander, "The Nightmare of Steroids," *Sports Illustrated,* 24 October 1988, p. 98.

17. *USA Today,* 6 April 1989, 2C.

18. Gabe Mirkin, "Hormonal Helpers," *Health,* March 1984, p. 6.

19. *American Journal of Nursing,* 86 (1986): 1217.

20. *Chicago Sun-Times,* 13 March 1989, p. A-12.

21. The *New York Times,* 21 November 1988, p. A22.

22. The Associated Press wire service reports, 7 December 1989.

23. Ibid.

Chapter Six
1. *Newsweek,* 10 October 1988, p. 57.

2. *Washington Post,* 18 June 1989, p. B10.

3. *USA Today,* 15 July 1986, p. 10A.

4. Ibid.

5. *USA Today,* 11 April 1989, p. 10A.

6. *The NCAA News,* 7 June 1989, p. 4.

7. *Physician and Sportsmedicine,* April 1988, p. 49.

8. *The NCAA News,* 2 August 1989, p. 2.

9. *The NCAA News,* 17 May 1989, 4.

10. *Journal of the American Medical Association,* 23 and 30 January 1987, p. 421.

11. *USA Today,* 20 June 1989, 1C.

12. Syndicated column by Mike Barnes, United Press International, as it appeared in *NCAA News,* 18 January 1989, p. 4.

13. Ibid.

14. *NCAA News, 2 August 1989, p. 2.*

15. *Newsweek,* 10 October 1988, p. 57.

16. *USA Today,* 15 June 1989, p. 9C.

17. *Newsweek,* 10 October 1988, p. 57.

18. *U.S. News & World Report,* 10 October 1988, p. 39.

19. *USA Today,* 18 November 1988, p. 11C.

20. The *New York Times,* 11 November 1988, p. D31.

21. *NCAA News,* 12 April 1989, p. 8.

22. *USA Today,* 6 April 1989, 10C.

23. United Press International as quoted in *NCAA News,* 2 August 1989, p. 2.

24. *NCAA News,* 2 August 1989, p. 2.

Afterword

1. Angela Patmore, *Sportsmen Under Stress* (London: Stanley Paul, 1986).

2. Associated Press wire story, 9 October 1988.

3. Fred Mitchell, "On the Bears" column, *Chicago Tribune,* 2 October 1988, p. 15.

4. *Chicago Sun-Times,* "Steroids: A Special Section," February 1989.

5. [Hammond] *Times,* 13 March 1989, p. A6.

6. William H. Lee, "On Nutrition," *American Druggist,* March 1987, p. 110.

BIBLIOGRAPHY

Newspapers and Magazines

Ann Arbor News
"Why Are Children Using Steroids?" February 27, 1989.

Chicago Sun-Times
"Jumbo-size Players Dominating the NFL." September 11, 1988.
"Steroids: A Special Section." February [no day given] 1989.

Daily News [New York]
"Steroids: Muscling in as a New Teen Menace." June 25, 1989.

Discover
"The Case Against Steroids." November 1983.
"Muscling in on Madness." September 1988.

Expo [Ball State University]
"Bulk Power." Spring 1986.

[Hammond] Times
"Coaches Warning Athletes," March 12, 1989.
"Steroids Lure Body Conscious," March 13, 1989.

"NCAA Members Face Need for Action," March 14, 1989.

Health
"Hormonal Helpers." March 1984.

Men's Fitness
"Steroid Punks." August 1988.
"Letters." August 1989.

Muncie Star
"Former Mr. Universe Arrested in Ohio on Steroids Charge." March 12, 1989

NCAA News
"Scott Says Steroid 'Black Eye' Unfair." January 18, 1989.
"IOC Removes Seven Drug-Testing Labs from Its Approved List." April 12, 1989.
"Team Sanctions for Positive Tests in Drug Program a Prominent Issue," May 19, 1989.
"Big Ten Coaches to Seek League Antisteroid Program," August 2, 1989.
"Steroid Abuse at Prep Level Is Target." August 2, 1989.

Newsweek
"The Insanity of Steroid Abuse." May 23, 1988.
"Using Chemistry to Get the Gold." July 25, 1989.
"The Doped-Up Games." October 10, 1988.

The *New York Times*
"Steroids in Sports." Five-part series. November 17–21, 1988.

Omni
"Dead Russian Athletes." March 1986.

Reader's Digest
"The Shocking Stain on International Athletics." August 1988.

Science
"The Drug of Champions." October 14, 1988.

Sporting News
"Drugs Remain Painful Subject for Rozelle." March 24, 1986.

Sports Illustrated
"Special Reports." January 21, 1985.
"Steroids: A Problem of Huge Dimensions." May 13, 1985.
"The NFL and Drugs: Fumbling for a Plan." February 10, 1986.
"An Athlete Disputes the Fairness of Mandatory Testing for Drugs." April 21, 1986.
"The Agony Must End." November 10, 1986.
"Reversing Field." December 8, 1986.
"Bosworth Faces the Music." January 5, 1987.
"A Former Husker 'Fesses Up." January 5, 1987.
"Consider the Risks." January 26, 1987.
"The Loser." October 3, 1988.
"The Nightmare of Steroids." October 24, 1988.
"Comrades." December 5, 1988.
"Steroids and the Young." December 26, 1988.
"The Death of an Athlete." February 20, 1989.

Time
"Shortcut to the Rambo Look." January 30, 1989.

USA Today
"The Debate: Drugs in Sports." July 15, 1986.
"Getting Strong, Getting Hurt: The Steroids Controversy." January 23, 1987.
"Swedish Doctor Defends Olympics Drug Testing." November 18, 1988.
"Policy Set on Steroids Testing." March 22, 1989.
"Chromium Picolinate." March 22, 1989.
"Soviet: Steroids Probe Is 'Positive.' " March 24, 1989.
"Steroids: Who's Blaming Whom?" April 6, 1989.
"Track Coach Tied to Steroids." April 6, 1989.
"Steroids Crackdown Would Be Real Abuse." April 11, 1989.
"Steroids: How Big a Problem in the NFL?" May 10, 1989.
"Doctor's Account Confirms Rumors." June 20, 1989.
" 'About 20' '84 Medalists Took Steroids." June 20, 1989.
"Ex-Steeler's Biggest Foe Now Is Time." July 5, 1989.
"Steroids Scandal." July 12, 1989.

"Steroids and AIDS." July 13, 1989.

"Steroids Founder Didn't Envision Use." August 1, 1989.

U.S. News & World Report

"A Game of Cat and Mouse." October 10, 1988.

Washington Post

"6.6% of Male 12th-Graders Say They Have Used Steroids." December 16, 1988.

"Senate Panel Told of Steroid Use in NFL." May 10, 1989.

"In Hue and Cry Over Steroids, Athletes Get Caught in the Middle." June 18, 1989.

Professional Journals

American Druggist

"There Are Nutritional Alternatives to Anabolic Steroids." March, 1987.

American Journal of Nursing

"The Weakness of Steroids." August 1986.

"Winning or Losing? Steroid Abuse in Athletes." November 1986.

American Journal of Sports Medicine

"Anabolic Steroids: A Review of the Literature." November 6, 1984.

Emergency Medicine

"Of Steroids and Sports." February 15, 1988.

Federation Proceedings

"Anabolic Steroids Are Fool's Gold." October 1981.

Health Education

"Preventing Steroid Abuse in Youth." August/September 1987.

Journal of the American Medical Association

"Anabolic Steroid Use and Perceived Effects in Ten Weight-Trained Women Athletes." May 17, 1985.

"Drug Testing and Moral Responsibility." November 1986.

"Steroids in Sports." January 23, 1987.

"Some Predict Increased Steroid Use in Sports Despite Drug Testing." June 12, 1987.

"Drug Abuse in Athletes." March 18, 1988.

"Issues of Drugs and Sports Gain Attention as Olympic Games Open in South Korea." September 16, 1988.
"Anabolic Steroid Use in Adolescence." Dec. 16, 1988.
"Estimated Prevalence of Anabolic Steroid Use Among Male High School Seniors. December 16, 1988.

Journal of Pediatric Health Care
"Androgenic-Anabolic Steroid Use in Adolescents." July/August 1989.

Physician & Sportsmedicine
"Side Effects of Anabolic Steroids in Weight-Trained Men." December 1983.
"Steroids Not Just for Athletes Anymore." June 1986.
"Drug Testing and Moral Responsibility." November 1986.
"Do Anabolic Steroids Pose an Ethical Dilemma for U.S. Physicians?" November 1986.
"NCAA Does Off-Season Testing for Steroids." April 1988.
"Gauging Steroid Use in High School Kids." August 1988.
"NCAA Documents Off-Season Steroid Use." November 1988.
"Cardiomyopathy and Cerebrovascular Accident Associated with Anabolic-Androgenic Steroid Use." Nov. 1988.

Scholastic Coach
"A.C.T.: The Steroid Alternative." January 1988.

Pamphlets
Anabolic Steroids and Athletes. American College of Sports Medicine. Undated.

Books
Berger, Gilda. *Drug Testing.* New York: Franklin Watts, 1987
Goldman, Bob. *Death in the Locker Room.* South Bend: Icarus Press, 1984
Patmore, Angela. *Sportsmen Under Stress.* London: Stanley Paul, 1986

Syndicated Columns
1989 Patricia McLaughlin/Universal Press Syndicate.

INDEX

121

ABOUT THE AUTHOR

Hank Nuwer, a contributing writer for *Inside Sports* and regular contributor to *Sport* magazine, has written profiles on dozens of college and professional athletes and coaches, including Wayman Tisdale, Chuck Person, Bill Walsh, Bobby Bowden, Ray Perkins, and Fred Akers. He once played first base for the Montreal Expos farm organization (on assignment).

Mr. Nuwer is married to Jenine Howard, a magazine editor, and has two sons.